POISON ON A PLATE

The Dangers in the Food We Eat
– and How to Avoid Them

Professor Richard Lacey

metro

First published simultaneously in hardback and paperback in Great Britain in 1998 by Metro Books (an imprint of Metro Publishing Limited), 19 Gerrard Street, London W1V 7LA

British Library Cataloguing in Publication Data. A CIP record of this book is available on request from the British Library.

Jacket design by Dave Farrow

ISBN 1 900512 46 7 (Hardback); 1 900512 45 9 (Paperback)

10 9 8 7 6 5 4 3 2 1

Typeset by Wakewing, High Wycombe
Printed in Great Britain by CPD Group, Wales

POISON ON A PLATE

By the same author

Safe Shopping, Safe Cooking, Safe Eating (Penguin, 1989)
Unfit for Human Consumption (Souvenir, 1991)
Hard to Swallow (Cambridge University Press, 1994)
Mad Cow Disease (Cypsela, 1994)
Red, Yellow and Blue Make White (Carlton Manor Publishing, 1997)

CONTENTS

INTRODUCTION

Towards the end of the 1980s, whilst Thatcherism was at its height and *laissez-faire* was the way of life in many spheres other than politics and economics, my quiet, comfortable and, I suppose, reasonably successful existence was about to come to an abrupt end. As both a doctor and a research scientist, fate had placed me at the epicentre of what was about to become a national obsession. My choice was simple. Should I toe the line and stay quiet? Or did my duties as both doctor and scientist demand that I speak out in the public good, at whatever cost to me and my family?

The problem which put me in such a painful dilemma was fundamental to daily life. I was being paid by the government to protect the public health. Yet day by day, I was growing more and more convinced that the government was allowing the public to be exposed to ever-more threatening and totally unacceptable health hazards from the most basic source of life: the food on our plates.

Over a thousand generations and more, mankind learned that, eaten under certain circumstances, some foods change from wholesome to poisonous. Early man, in my opinion, learned to use fire for cooking not merely to change food's flavour but to make food safer: he probably did not understand why – the fact that the heat involved in cooking killed many harmful bacteria was unknown to him – but over many centuries he must have noticed that fewer people fell ill after eating cooked food, and in particular meat, than after they ate it raw. Similarly, many ancient religions forbid certain eating practices but, I would suggest, such prohibitions came about as much for reasons of public health than those of religious faith: eating pork, for instance, was banned by early Judaism and later by Islam, which was in fact very good public health law in areas of warm climate before the days of refrigeration. Thus man developed ways of protecting himself from food poisoning. But in the mid-1980s, from my post of Professor of Microbiology at Leeds

University, I was experiencing growing concern that such wisdom of the centuries was being dumped in favour of that icon of Thatcherite Britain: profit.

Since the 1960s, the British lifestyle had changed almost beyond recognition from my childhood in the immediate postwar years. More and more married women were going out to work which, of course, gave them less time to cook the traditional meals their housewife mothers had served. The manufacturers of household appliances were quick to spot marketing opportunities this social change brought: the microwave oven and the deep-freeze, for instance, were soon to become standard items in most homes.

In the British countryside, things were changing, too. Traditional farming methods were being forgotten as farmers were urged on to even higher productivity (despite the fact that, in Europe at least, we were stockpiling huge amounts of unwanted produce). Food production was being boosted by more intensive methods, farm animals were having injected a wide range of chemical and hormone boosters, and, almost unnoticed, millions of years of feeding habits were being changed: that humble herbivore, the cow, was being forced into becoming a carnivore by being fed discarded and otherwise unusable animal remains.

The development of kitchen appliances and techniques in the preparation of food, and the changes in farming methods, represented progress in the eyes of most people. In other eyes, it represented profit. To me and a handful of other scientists, it represented something far worse. In casting aside the hard-won experience of the ages we were in fact regressing, going backwards in time and endangering society. Someone, somewhere, had to speak out. By accident more than design, that person turned out to be me.

Part One

WHISTLE-BLOWING

1

DEATH OF A TEENAGER

He stood six feet seven inches and weighed more than 16 stone. At school, he had played rugby and on leaving kept up his passion for ice-skating. He had dozens of close friends and hundreds of acquaintances, and many of them called him The Lampost. 'Not because he was so tall,' one of those girlfriends was to say tearfully later, 'but because you could lean on him when you had troubles. He was that sort of lad, someone you could always turn to for advice or a few words of comfort.'

Young Matthew Parker grew up in an area of South Yorkshire whose traditional industries, coal and the railways, had been devastated after privatization. When he took five good GSEs at the local comprehensive school in Armthorpe, near Doncaster, both his parents and his teachers wanted him to stay on to do A levels and aim for university. But Matthew had ambitions of his own, inspired by his uncle Alan, a globe-trotting chef whose culinary skills had allowed him to pursue his trade in many parts of the world: at present, Alan is a chef at the American Embassy in Bonn.

Like most teenagers, Matthew enjoyed his food. For a youth of his size, it was not surprising that he wolfed down any meal that was put in front of him and many more that he bought from various fast-food restaurants after an evening out: burgers, pies, curries, pizzas, fish and chips, the sort of food that is the staple part of a million teenage diets. At home, his mother cooked him meals like cottage pie and spaghetti Bolognaise from minced beef and always insisted that he and his brother Russell also had plenty of fruit and fresh vegetables. For young, strong, active lads, this diet combined the calories they needed for energy with the vitamins and roughage that their social-worker mother Doreen Parker thought would stand them in good stead in later life. Matthew, as they say in South Yorkshire, was 'as fit as a lop'.

No one knew that food, which Matthew wanted to make the centrepiece of his working life, would be the cause of his tragically young death.

He left school at 16 and enlisted on a catering course at the local technical college. In an area where thousands of youngsters have little hope of a decent job, he began to work in local pubs and clubs, earning a good wage for a youth of his age. After work, there were nights out with his mates, often finishing at a burger bar or a kebab house. Inevitably for a lad of his good looks and physical presence, there was a stream of girlfriends. Eventually, he seemed to settle with one particular lass, and his mother, who had by now gone through a divorce, was pleased that her oldest son seemed set fair for a good job, marriage, a nice home and, later perhaps, children.

When it began to go wrong, no one really noticed. At first, Matthew suddenly gave up his interest in cooking and took a mundane job in a local factory. At about the same time, he and his steady girlfriend parted company. Matthew was now living with his father, John, who had remarried, and Doreen began to hear reports that her son was becoming moody, sitting alone in the works canteen, ignoring his old friends. Some of those friends called on Doreen to express their concern, but she brushed it aside. As a woman who works with troubled teenagers in a residential home, she put it down to the after-effects of Matthew's broken romance. 'Most parents know just how sulky and withdrawn teenagers can be from time to time,' she recalls now. It was, she thought, just a passing phase…

Then she began to hear that Matthew had been staggering about in the streets. This was much more worrying, especially in a small, tight-knit community like Armthorpe, where everyone knows everyone else and gossip travels quickly. Matthew, she assumed, had begun to drink heavily. Even worse, she feared that her son had taken to drugs. When asked, Matthew vehemently denied using drugs. But he did admit he was worried because he was suffering considerable pain in his legs.

For the first time, the family began to worry that something was seriously amiss. But when they first sought medical advice, they were told: 'Matthew is just suffering from growing pains.' Recalling that diagnosis, Doreen still winces: 'Growing pains! In a lad who was already six feet seven? For the first time, I began to worry about the efficiency of the medical profession.'

As December came in 1996, a cousin who worked in the local branch of Sainsbury's saw Matthew stagger into the store at 9.30a.m. and assumed that he was either very drunk or under the influence of drugs.

Then, on 7 December 1996, Matthew went Christmas shopping with his father. Without warning, he began to stagger uncontrollably, swaying from side to side in danger of crashing into the piled displays of Christmas goods. Other shoppers, assuming that this tall young man was drunk, glared and muttered their disapproval. John, knowing that his son had not taken a single drink, was too alarmed to be embarrassed. This was something strange and very mysterious, behaviour he had never witnessed before in any human being. Wracked with worry, he took his distressed son to the emergency unit at the Doncaster Royal Infirmary.

Medical staff did what tests they could to identify the illness. The following day, they gave Matthew a brain scan – a CAT scan – and his anxious family waited for the results. It was the first time that his father and mother had met since their divorce. With them, the whole family, including John's new wife, Doreen's father, and Matthew's uncles and aunts were gathered together, as is the way of people in mining communities, who have long lived with the dread of disaster. After what seemed like hours, the consultant neurologist asked to see the parents in private.

'Have you ever heard of Creutzfeldt-Jakob disease?' the consultant asked quietly.

'Never,' they both replied, mystified.

The consultant paused. 'Well, have you heard of Mad Cow Disease?'

It took a while to sink in. Doreen, like most people in Britain at the time, had read newspaper reports, which described a disease that earned its tabloid press name because its cattle victims do literally go mad: they prance about in uncontrollable movements like a bucking bronco trying to unseat an invisible rider, or they butt their heads furiously against a wall or a tree – until they lose the use of their legs altogether and fall down. And she had seen the films on television of cows suffering from it. But, also like most people in Britain, she had dismissed it as yet another food scare story of the type which had come and gone with regularity during the 1990s. Yes, she knew that some cows had gone mad but what did that have to do with her son?

'Well, I'm afraid that your son could be suffering from the human equivalent which we call new-variant CJD. It seems to affect young people.'

Ever since she had known that Matthew was to have a CAT scan, Doreen had persuaded herself that her son might have a brain tumour. Although she knew such a condition was highly dangerous, she also knew that some tumours can be benign and that others can be cured either by surgery or chemotherapy. At least such a diagnosis would have been one she understood, and that offered Matthew some hope. To be faced now with a diagnosis that she did not understand, without being told of any hope of recovery, was extremely alarming. Needing reassurance, Doreen asked if her father, Matthew Burn, for whom the teenager had been named, could be brought into the meeting. As it happened, Mr Burn had been taking a keen interest in the Mad Cow epidemic and had read all the newspaper stories he could find.

'The doctor repeated what he had told us and and I could see immediately from the look on Dad's face that the condition was terminal,' says Doreen. What hope she had had begun to ebb away.

Matthew was transferred immediately to the Royal Hallamshire Hospital in Sheffield, which they were told had better facilities and a medical staff more experienced in dealing with rare brain disorders. There the family's hope was restored: doctors in Sheffield reassured them that whatever Matthew was suffering from, it was not CJD.

'That sent my spirits soaring,' says Doreen. But as Christmas approached and the family made the arduous daily journey to Sheffield and back, the fact that Matthew did not have CJD brought little consolation, especially as no other diagnosis was forthcoming, and as his condition worsened their hopes receded. They were told that Matthew could have this disease, then that disease, none of which were familiar. And, perplexingly, hospital officials told them on several separate occasions 'It is not CJD so don't go to the tabloid press.'

'I didn't pay much attention to this in the beginning because I was so delighted that Matthew didn't have the disease that I pushed awkward questions to the back of my mind,' says Doreen. 'But then I began to realise that there was a contradiction here. The thought of going to the press had never crossed my mind but why was the hospital so worried about it? After all, if I were to ring up some reporter and tell him that my son *didn't* have CJD, he would tell me to stop wasting his time. People who *don't* have rare diseases don't make stories, do they?'

Christmas 1996 was a nightmare time for Matthew's family. Almost every day, Doreen made the long journey to Sheffield only to see her son's condition deteriorate. On the days she did not go, Matthew's father or other relatives made the trip: at every visiting time, his bed was surrounded by friends and family. His legs pains began to worsen and then he began to lose his voice. He needed a catheter to pass urine, which he hated, and slowly but surely his ability to swallow began to fade. He began to be able to drink only by taking tiny sips from a glass. Then he used a straw. As the condition worsened, the straw was replaced by a baby's feeder cup. Eventually, he was fed by drip feed and the only way he could take liquids was through a large syringe.

But still the family did not know what was wrong. The hospital continued with a series of exhaustive tests including two lumbar punctures and a skin biopsy. Several theories were posed and then abandoned. As Christmas approached, the family agreed that Matthew should go home for a few days. It took a wheelchair and four men to get him into Doreen's semi, where she had made up his bed in the lounge. His friends came in their dozens – 'It was like a youth club in here,' says Doreen – but he was oblivious to them. The television was placed at the foot of his bed but even when his favourite programmes came on, he stared blankly into space.

Doreen slept on the settee by his bedside, snatching a few minutes rest here and there. One morning, she woke at 4a.m. to find Matthew thrashing about on the floor. It took her several hours to get him back into bed, for he was by now unable to move his once-muscular body himself. To this day, she does not know how he had managed to get out of bed. But it is likely that the most terrible symptoms of his illness had struck: hallucinations.

After Christmas, Matthew went back to hospital and the tests went on. It was, says Doreen, the worst six weeks of the family agony for now the hallucinations were becoming ever-more terrifying. One day, he asked his mother to take him home because he was late for school. On another, he believed that the man in the bed opposite had given birth to a baby during the night. Sometimes, the hallucinations drove Matthew to violence: he punched a hole in the plasterboard wall of his hospital ward. He tore down the curtains from the window by his bed and then lay sucking a corner of the curtain material as a comforter.

'It was as though he wanted a dummy,' says Doreen. 'He seemed to have regressed in three short months from a fine, strong young man back through his school days until he was a babe-in-arms again. By this time, he couldn't speak at all. He pointed at things and made gestures that, for instance, he wanted his hurting legs massaged, a job his grandfather always did. We all had jobs: I held his hand and spoke to him in the way a mother speaks to her baby. When his brother Russell visited, Matthew would take food on a spoon only from him.'

Halfway through February, the doctors decided on one final test: a brain biopsy, which means the surgical removal of a small sample of brain tissue for microscopic examination, a procedure undertaken only in the most severe of cases. Finally, on 14 February, a doctor took Doreen and John aside and confessed that they had been wrong: the brain biopsy had proved that Matthew had new-variant CJD. And, he said gravely, the condition was terminal.

Recalling this moment, Doreen's tears give way to a barely suppressed anger: 'Why did they wait so long to tell us? They said he didn't have CJD, but they must have come to suspect it. Was it because they were terrified of admitting that there was another new-variant CJD case, because it would have meant meant more stories in the newspapers? I don't know their reasoning but we had been put through ten weeks of absolute hell, given false hope after, back before Christmas, we had been told in Doncaster that all hope was gone. Had they left it there, we could have come to terms with the awfulness of it all and had a few weeks of quality time with Matthew. I will never, ever, forgive them for that.'

Matthew Parker, aged 19, died at 4.50p.m. on Sunday 23 March 1997, in a nursing home near his South Yorkshire home. All his family had been around his bedside since the early hours of the day. His grandfather had been massaging his pain-wracked legs when they began to turn blue. His mother, holding his hand, watched the flesh turn blue in her grasp a few minutes later. But he was still breathing. His brother, Russell, two years younger, had been at the bedside throughout the day. He could no longer bear the sadness so he wished his unconscious brother farewell and left. Fifteen minutes later, Matthew died.

'I am sure he held on until Russell left,' says their mother. 'He did not want to die in front of his brother.'

On 20 August 1997, the Doncaster Deputy Coroner, Fred Curtis, recorded a verdict of death by misadventure on Matthew Parker and stated that 'on the balance of probabilities' he had contracted new-variant CJD as a result of eating beef infected with Bovine Spongiform Encephalopathy – BSE, known popularly as Mad Cow Disease. He was the twenty-second young person in Britain known to have contracted the disease.

CJD is just one of a number of diseases – including infections caused by listeria, salmonella and *E. coli* – that, in recent years, have been arriving on our plates in the food we eat with increasing regularity. I suspect that many members of the public dismiss the many food-poisoning crises reported in the press as scare stories. But for those who are struck down by these illnesses they are far from that. The diseases are not all inevitably fatal, like CJD, but all cause suffering and may in some cases cause death. Given proper thought, preventive measures and food-handling procedures, they are preventable.

Or they would have been, had not the government of recent decades, in its handling of such crises, failed repeatedly – as I shall show – in its duty to protect the health and the wellbeing of the people it represents. As a result, many have suffered unnecessarily. In the case of CJD, the most severe and the most mismanaged crisis of all, hundreds or even thousands of Britons may already be infected with it, doomed unnecessarily. Matthew Parker, and others like him, need not have died.

Because of my chosen career, I have specialist knowledge of these diseases and was to find myself involved in many cases of outbreaks of them. In the face of such chilling facts I found it necessary, despite the personal cost, to speak out about them. The facts behind these diseases, and the story of these crises and my involvement with them, are what this book is about.

2

EARLY ENCOUNTERS

My involvement in food-poisoning crises came about in part because of my unusual crossover of knowledge. There is a tendency for the majority of modern doctors to follow a well-defined path towards medical specialization, resulting in a career either as a hospital consultant or perhaps as a teacher at medical college, and it is unusual for someone to pursue careers in both medicine and science. However, although I trained as a doctor, from an early age I was determined to share science – and, in particular, scientific research – with medicine. While I trained, I spread my interests in science, too, so that I had skills in what might be termed 'hands-on' experience in fighting existing outbreaks of disease by laboratory analysis, and also in pure research, aimed at finding the cause of other diseases and leading, hopefully, to a cure for such diseases. As well as an MB in medicine, I also took an MA in biochemistry and later a BCh in surgery. (I went on from there, eventually, to have an MD in microbiology, a PhD in genetics at Bristol University and a Diploma in Child Health, and to become a Fellow of the Royal College of Surgeons.) After an unsatisfying period as a junior doctor at the London Hospital in Whitechapel, I decided that my future in medicine would be in research rather than in direct contact with the patient.

By the late 1960s, when I began my career in research, the international pharmaceutical industry, which includes some of the biggest, wealthiest and most powerful companies in the world, was coming more and more under the spotlight of public scrutiny. In the immediate postwar years, science had been hailed as the panacea for all the ills of the human race. Antibiotics had become widely available, in the Western world at least, and great strides had been made in the treatment of diseases that had once killed millions of people every year: tuberculosis, smallpox, diphtheria, typhoid and many more fell under the control of man, at least in areas where these new drugs and vaccines were available. Science, too, was powering important advances in agriculture, which were bringing about huge increases in productivity, both in crops and in farm livestock. Some optimistic commentators were beginning to hail the age where disease and starvation were to be banished from the surface of the Earth for ever.

There had, indeed, been many advances of enormous importance and it is not my intention to decry them: science has in the past 50 years taken some of the most important strides forward in the history of the human race. Many, many millions of people are alive today who would otherwise have died prematurely from disease, hunger and poverty or a deadly combination of all three. However, people's attitudes were beginning to change. Some scientists began to show concern that, in no small number of cases, these so-called advances had gone a stride too far: in this rush towards a science-driven utopia, drugs and chemicals had been released on the public or into the environment that had not been properly and thoroughly tested, their long-term effects on the world in which we live either overlooked or simply ignored.

Then cracks began to show in the chemical-pharmaceutical industry's suit of shining armour. First, there was the DDT disaster, in which vast quantities of this persistent and highly toxic chemical were allowed to be sprayed on crops as a pesticide throughout the world. In America, one of the first great prophets of the environmental movement, Rachel Carson, demonstrated the possible effects of this in a seminal book called *Silent Spring*, in which she painted a picture of the Earth devoid of birds, butterflies and many other creatures, because they had all been poisoned by artificial pesticides. Medical researches caused increasing concern by showing that these pesticides were evident in the fetuses of stillborn or deformed children, particularly in the Third World, where DDT and similar pesticides had been used in vast quantities to combat disease-carrying insects like the mosquito and the tsetse fly. DDT was traced in the sterile eggs of penguins in Antarctica; and in Britain in the early 1960s, ornithologists studying a sudden plunge in the numbers of birds of prey discovered large quantities of three sinister chemicals in the sterile eggs of many species of hawks: aldrin, dieldrin and heptachlor. These chemicals were found to have come from pesticide dressings used by farmers on cereal crops. Corn is, of course, a staple part of the diet of many species of songbirds, and tests had shown that, in the tiny quantities involved, these smaller birds suffered little harm. What no one had investigated was what happened to those pesticides in the songbird physiology. Further investigation showed that the songbirds were storing these poisons in their livers. When hawks ate these prey species, the poisons were also stored in their livers in ever-greater proportions and eventually invaded their reproductive systems. The effects drove many to the point of extinction before the government banned the use of aldrin, dieldrin and heptachlor.

This case created widespread condemnation from country-lovers and bewilderment and distress to many farmers, who were accused of poisoning the countryside in the search for greater productivity. But it is important to point out that farmers were not to blame. They were, and still are to a lesser extent, under pressure from the government to increase production, so as to lessen the flow of imported food into Britain, which is a continual strain on the balance of payments. They had been offered pesticides by reputable agri-chemical companies to stop insect damage to their cereal crops and had used them in good faith; they were farmers, after all, not biochemists, and any damaging side effects should have been taken into account by the researchers who developed and tested these products for the manufacturers. Patently, this was not done; but even so, in the public mind at least, it was the farmers, not the scientists, who stood in the front line of condemnation.

Serious as the DDT poisoning was, however, it pertained only to animals and humans in the Third World, and it passed without notice amongst the majority of Britain's urban population. Then came a disaster that affected human beings in Britain itself: thalidomide. Thalidomide was a drug which suppressed vomiting, one of the more unpleasant side effects of pregnancy, and had been widely prescribed to pregnant mothers by doctors who, at the beginning at least, had no idea of its toxicity. Then babies began to be born with horrific deformities, such as missing arms and legs. It soon struck home to everyone in the scientific community that the governments involved for many years afterward did everything possible to cover up the implications of this medical disaster. But for the courage of the *Sunday Times*, which conducted an outspoken campaign, it is likely that thalidomide victims would have remained uncompensated to this day – though, of course, there can never be adequate compensation for such suffering.

The aftermath of the thalidomide affair had an important effect on my own career. In 1968, Harold Wilson's Labour government introduced the Medicines Act, which, still in force today, was an attempt by the government to force pharmaceutical companies to test all active ingredients in any drugs put on the market and to prove beyond scientific doubt that they could have no long-term side effects. This was a significant step forward because, until then, drug manufacturers had primarily to show only that their products were effective in treating a certain condition, and they had less obligation to guarantee safety. Now, unless they could demonstrate that all components of any compound were harmless in other ways, a new drug could not be marketed. In other words, the onus was placed fair and square on the industry's scientists. This requirement, which to the layman must seem to be so obviously essential as to be unnecessary to enforce legally on any reputable manufacturer, meant that the drug companies had to launch enormously costly and time-consuming trials, first on animals and then on human volunteers. This exhaustive process can add years to the introduction of a new drug.

The very year that the Medicines Act was introduced was also the year when I took my first step into pure research, when I became lecturer and then reader in Clinical Microbiology at the University of Bristol. These were halcyon days for medical research, for Wilson had promised to modernize Britain 'in the white heat of technology', and there were funds available which allowed university academics to carry out extensive research alongside their teaching duties.

My role became one of an independent scientist working for the good of the public health. It included many aspects – for instance, I researched and campaigned (with eventual success) against the use of a commonly prescribed antibiotic marketed under the name of Septrin – but a large part of my work was concerned with bacteria.

Bacteria have, over the years, had a bad press. Words like *germs*, *microbes* and *bacteria* are associated in the public mind with dirt, illness and even death. This is by and large unfair, for there are many, many thousands of types of bacteria in existence and some millions of germs in the healthy human body. Most of them do important work for us in helping us digest our food, for instance, making vitamins, or attacking harmful micro-organisms.

There are other bacteria, however, such as the various types of salmonella and listeria, which can and do cause serious illness amongst humans. They cause severe intestinal pain, and chronic diarrhoea which can lead to blood loss, the draining away of vital body salts and, in extreme cases, high levels of dehydration. For all victims, this is extremely unpleasant. For the vulnerable, such as the very young, the old, those already in ill health and pregnant women, it can mean death. These bacteria, often called 'killer bugs' by the tabloid press, usually come from animals which we eat although, in some cases, they are not dangerous to the host animal. This makes it particularly difficult for doctors and microbiologists to persuade farmers or intensive poultry producers that something is wrong: if their animals or chickens are perfectly healthy, they argue, how can they pass on disease in their meat or eggs?

The study of microbiology is a relatively new science. It was made possible by methods of growing bacterium cultures under laboratory conditions on dishes of nutrient jelly, the technique by which Sir Alexander Fleming discovered penicillin, one of the historic medical breakthroughs, by accident in 1928. When he left a culture of staphylococcus, a potentially dangerous bacterium, exposed to the air, stray spores of the mould *Penicillium* floated in through the lab window and began to attack the bacteria. Like many a British scientist before and since, he did very little to exploit this major advance in medical science. It was not until World War Two, when penicillin secrets were given to the Americans, that its mass exploitation began, mainly as a treatment for wounded troops. Penicillin, named the 'magic bullet' by the press, and various other antibiotics developed from it, did not become widely available to the general public until the late 1940s.

The term magic bullet well describes the best quality of antibiotics, which can kill dangerous bacteria invading the human body without damaging other, beneficial, organisms. Penicillin and major advances in medical technology, such as the invention of the electron microscope, added considerable impetus to the race to control disease bacteria.

A significant episode in bacterial research was a series of experiments begun by American doctors in the 1940s, using what would now be considered ethically suspect methods. They gave volunteer black prison convicts controlled doses of salmonella bacteria to see how much they could consume before they became ill. Presumably, these unfortunate blacks were offered some easing of their prison conditions in return for the cooperation. Unfortunately, the entire trial was based on bad science, and it set back the cause of bacterial research for the best part of 40 years. The salmonella doses were delivered to the prisoners in ever growing concentrations in water, which was not judged to be of any importance at the time. The conclusion was that to become ill, a victim must ingest some 100,000 bacteria. This may seems like a very large number, but a single bacterium is so small that such a number packed tightly together would be invisible to the human eye: some ten million would fit onto a pinhead. To find 100,000 in a single portion of food would be extremely unusual, unless the food had been so badly prepared as to be virtually inedible. This 100,000 figure became established throughout the medical world and the risks of serious illness or even death from salmonella poisoning were perceived to be relatively minor, particularly in the Western world, where food hygiene and storage practices were judged to be of high quality.

Then in the 1970s and 1980s came two serious outbreaks which sent the microbiologists back to the drawing board. One involved a brand of chocolate called Rocky, manufactured in Italy, and the second Cheddar cheese. Many hundreds of people became ill in the United Kingdom and in Canada, where the cheese had been eaten. Distressing as this was for the victims, it proved a bonus for medical science, for in each case there were samples of infected food left behind which could be used for analysis – a rare opportunity for, in most cases of food poisoning, the food itself has been consumed completely and therefore destroyed in the victims' stomachs and intestines.

Cheese and chocolate samples were broken down into laboratory specimens to grow cultures which were thoroughly examined. Suddenly, received wisdom was turned on its head. It was discovered that, when ingested in a fatty substance, such as cheese or chocolate, harmful bacteria have a much greater chance of survival from attack by the human body's natural defence mechanisms, such as stomach acids and beneficial bacteria, than when ingested in water, as in the 1940s American experiments with black convicts. The fat in the food provides the harmful bacteria with a protective shield, under which they can multiply at enormous speed in the gut, growing so fast that they overwhelm the natural defences.

Most significantly, the study showed that, ingested with fat, as few as ten salmonella bacteria can cause serious disease, a finding which divided the accepted figure by *ten thousand*. A fundamental flaw in the original American study was exposed: those volunteers had taken their poison with water but, in real life, that would be an extremely unlikely event because, in the West at least, water is rarely contaminated to that extent. Food, and badly prepared food in particular, is a much more likely carrier for harmful bacteria and as most foods except boiled vegetables contain some fat, they also provide the invaders with their own built-in defence system.

Crucial to the significance of these findings is the rate at which harmful bacteria multiply inside the body. Most food-poisoning cases take between 12 and 36 hours to develop, an extremely short incubation period. The reason for this is the speed at which these bacteria can multiply, doubling their numbers three times an hour until the body can cope with no more. The following rough calculation table may illustrate this:

Multiplication rates of a single *Salmonella enteritidis* bacterium from poultry, which grows like an amoeba, by splitting itself into two independent organisms every 20 minutes:

20 minutes:	2
40 minutes:	4
One hour:	8
Two hours:	64
Three hours:	512
Four hours:	4,000
Five hours:	32,000
Six hours:	250,000
Seven hours:	2,000,000
Eight hours:	16,000,000
Nine hours:	120,000,000
Ten hours:	1,000,000,000

These figures represent the potential harm that can be done by a single bacterium once the bacteria have entered the human body. In the early stages at least, some of these bacteria will fall victim to the body's natural defences, such as enzymes in the pancreas which eat bacteria and thrive on it, or stomach acid. There are hundreds of millions of these helpful bacteria in the normal healthy body, but even they cannot cope with the explosive growth of the most harmful bacteria such as salmonella once it takes hold, and even modern medicines like antibiotics do not help – indeed, they may cause the salmonella to persist. In a body which is not so healthy, or whose defence resources have been divided as in pregnant women, even the replacement of fluids lost as a result of the infection can sometimes come too late. For newborn babies, the threat cannot be over-exaggerated because they are born without any natural defence mechanisms at all. They have to obtain their helpful bacteria from their mothers, usually through touch. Once ingested these, too, will multiply at enormous speed to give the youngster the protection it must have, unless the harmful ones get there first and tragedy strikes.

As the science of microbiology and its related disciplines were beginning to learn these painful lessons, it became increasingly obvious that the most successful way of preventing acute food poisoning was to prevent harmful bacteria getting into food in the first place. Or, if it was already there, to kill it by proper cooking. The trouble was that changes in methods of storing and cooking food were making this more difficult, as I was to discover.

3

OUTBREAK

In 1983, after ten years as Consultant in Infectious Diseases with the East Anglian Health Authority, where I had expanded my research into antibiotics, I was appointed Professor of Medical Microbiology at Leeds University. This was an unusual type of appointment in the United Kingdom because I had, in fact, two bosses. The post was funded up to 40 per cent by the University, for which I lectured and continued my research, and the remaining 60 per cent came from the National Health Service (NHS), for which I ran the diagnostic laboratory and became Infectious Disease Officer at Leeds General Infirmary, one of Britain's leading teaching hospitals. It was, for me, an ideal post because it combined all my training as a doctor with laboratory analysis and pure research, which was now moving into the field of food poisoning.

As a professor, I had – or thought I had – *tenure,* that centuries-old English academic status, which meant that I could not be sacked except for gross personal misconduct. Quite what the latter means is difficult to establish, but presumably it would include becoming an alcoholic, a drug addict, or a relentless seducer of undergraduates. So long as I did not fall foul of such personal foibles, tenure gave me the right to continue my research and publish any findings that resulted, however controversial or upsetting to various political or industrial interests, without fear of losing my job. This was why tenure was established: to encourage academic freedom to flourish.

In the early 1980s, microbiology – the study of microscopic living organisms – was not a widespread discipline in the health service. This was partly because it was new, and partly because the necessary laboratory equipment and skilled staff required to operate it were expensive. However, as the spread of disease by bacteria or viruses began to be more fully understood, microbiology became – and continues to be – more and more vital. In hospitals, the presence of vulnerable patients makes it critically important to prevent the spread of disease from one patient to another and, indeed, to the medical and auxiliary staff. In appointing me, Leeds had decided to use the new weapons science was making available.

Other health authorities in the North of England had not yet taken such a step, including the one responsible for Wakefield, the West Yorkshire city a few miles south of Leeds. In 1984 Wakefield Health Authority asked me if I would act for them as an honorary Consultant Microbiologist. I accepted in principle, but there had to be negotiations between Wakefield and my Leeds employers. As is the way of these things, the red tape began to tangle and negotiations were not concluded before disaster struck.

Stanley Royd Hospital in Wakefield was an archetypal example of many such institutions in Britain, built in the nineteenth century as a lunatic asylum. It was an extremely difficult building to maintain: too big in some ways, too small in others, with echoing wards and a catering system that owed more to a grand country house than an institution dedicated to the care of the sick. Although money had been spent on modern medical and surgical equipment, and although its dispensary was equipped with all the latest drugs, its one big kitchen had been subject to years of neglect.

The kitchen was very old, furnished with catering equipment that was inadequate and almost as tatty as the building, and remote from most of the wards. The catering staff were badly paid and, as an official report was later to point out, badly trained and managed; morale was low. The food, I later learned, was awful. Much of it was prepared hours in advance and then trundled down long corridors on trolleys to the wards where, as often as not, it waited even longer before it was dished up to the patients. It was as though no one in the place had ever been told that one of the most common ways for human beings to contract disease is in the food they eat, and that it is difficult to find a better breeding ground for dangerous bacteria than lukewarm food left standing for several hours.

The hospital staff might have been more alert had they known that, earlier in that year, 1984, there had already been one major food-poisoning outbreak in Britain – or rather on aircraft flying from Britain to the United States. In this case, 766 people using British Airways flights had suffered severe bouts of poisoning by *Salmonella enteritidis*, a type of the bacteria common in eggs and poultry. This is one of those strains of bacteria that is particularly difficult to combat because, although it can cause very severe illness indeed in human beings, it rarely harms the poultry which are its hosts. Had this fact become known to the public and, in particular, to politicians at the time of the British Airways outbreak, many subsequent problems could have been avoided; however, it did not, because the outbreak was hushed up by anxious British Airways public-relations staff who, understandably at a time when long-haul airlines were making much of the quality of the food they served, did not wish the travelling public to know that their food had killed two people and caused serious distress to hundreds more. If the media did get hold of the story, little was made of it: food poisoning was not yet a big story. That state of affairs was about to change for ever.

Over the late-summer bank holiday weekend at the end of August 1984, there was a major heat wave. At the Stanley Royd hospital in Wakefield, patients sweltered in the wards and, in the ancient kitchen, temperatures must have been nigh on unbearable – for all professional kitchens, even in relatively small restaurants, begin to resemble Dante's Inferno at peak cooking times. As the Stanley Royd catering staff laboured hard to feed many hundreds of mouths, the heat exacerbated the already poor conditions of food preparation.

As the holiday weekend passed, doctors and nursing staff were alarmed when people already mentally sick began to complain of intense intestinal pains. Within 24 hours, *S. typhimurium*, another particularly nasty salmonella bug, had spread like wildfire round the wards. It became obvious that a major medical emergency was underway. Then people began to die. As the death toll climbed towards ten, then a dozen, patients and their relatives began to demand that patients should be moved. Some even argued that the hospital should be completely evacuated.

The story was reported by local and national media, and I read all this with growing anxiety from my laboratory in Leeds, only 12 miles or so away, expecting the phone to ring. Nothing happened. For, although it had been agreed that I should take over as honorary consultant to the Wakefield Hospital Authority the following 1 January, that was still four months away. And bureaucracy being what it is, someone, somewhere, decided that the hospital could manage the crisis without the best equipped and most modern microbiology laboratory for many miles. By the time the outbreak began to subside, 455 patients and staff had suffered severe salmonella poisoning and 19 patients, mainly elderly, had died.

A public enquiry was ordered, and the investigations were underway when I finally took over my post as Consultant Microbiologist. One of the major responsibilities in our new brief was to advise on future catering arrangements in the hope of preventing similar outbreaks. One of my first acts was to tour the Stanley Royd kitchen and inspect the catering system. I was appalled to see the poor conditions. The major problem, as I saw it, was the extended time between food being prepared and cooked, and being served. Food was routinely left standing in a lukewarm state for up to two hours or more. The risk of food developing dangerous bacterial colonies, and the fact that the August heat had magnified this danger, should have been obvious to even the lowliest members of a professional catering operation, never mind the hospital medical staff. Unfortunately, I was not able to give this evidence to the enquiry because I had not taken up my post at the time of the events.

Even in so-called Third World countries, people have understood the dangers of high temperatures for centuries: in hot countries, most meat is cooked within hours of being obtained, and then served piping hot. Though it may seem cruel to Western eyes, in places where there is no refrigeration in Asia and Africa, poultry is sold live in local markets so that it can be slaughtered and prepared by the cook within minutes, or at the most an hour or so, of death. They know that food, and particularly meat, left lying around in hot climates can become dangerous if not actually lethal. One presumes this fact was well known to the authorities at Stanley Royd. If so, it appears to have been ignored.

My idea then, and now, for the best way of preventing such outbreaks in hospitals or similar institutions is that initial preparation should take place in a central kitchen but that the final cooking process should take place, at temperatures high enough to kill bacteria of the salmonella or listeria types, at the point of service: i.e. near the hospital ward. This, of course, would mean additional catering staff and expensive cooking equipment being installed in the wards. But when the Stanley Royd outbreak occurred, government policy was imposing large cuts in public spending. The Wakefield Health Authority was looking for ways of saving money, not spending more, and such an ideal solution was hardly on the cards.

The public enquiry took a year to report. It produced an extremely lengthy document that, in my opinion, virtually ignored the underlying causes of the disaster. The poisoning, it suggested, had been caused by beef which had been cooked the day before serving, sliced, and left to lie around all night and the following morning in already warm conditions which were exacerbated by the heat wave. The enquiry report concluded by blaming 'catering errors' set against a background of 'inadequate management', as though the staff themselves were to blame for the Victorian conditions of their workplace and the hopelessly inadequate procedures for delivering meals to patients.

It was a highly unsatisfactory conclusion to a grave emergency. But it did not stop there. Within weeks of the report, without any consultation whatsoever with myself or members of the clinical staff, Wakefield Health Authority issued an announcement which I still find totally inexplicable more than a decade later. As a result of the report, the authority had decided to institute a cook-chill policy, under which food would be prepared and cooked several days before serving, chilled and then sent back to the original kitchens at Stanley Royd to be reheated and distributed in the same old way.

The main thrust of the enquiry report had been that the times between cooking and serving should be substantially reduced. Yet here was a plan that would extend that time, not by a few hours, but by days. What's more, the cook-chill process was already coming under investigation by many microbiologists, including myself; concerned about the lack of published evaluation for it and the theoretical dangers, we perceived it as a major new threat to public health. As long ago as 1970, the then Department of Health and Social Security (DHSS), now split up, warned that cook-chill catering was not a safe method of feeding a community, because of the risk of bacterial contamination. It was cook-chill techniques that were the major suspect for causing the British Airways salmonella outbreak.

I will go into the dangers of cook-chill in more scientific detail in chapter four. Suffice it to say here that it is a technique very different from and far less satisfactory than the better-known deep-freezing. Providing that deep-frozen food has been hygienically prepared before going into a deep-freeze, and is thoroughly cooked all the way through after being properly defrosted, it is quite safe (although, sadly, these conditions are all too often inadequately met). Cook-chill, however, never freezes the food totally and all too often leaves it in that potentially lethal lukewarm state where certain types of bacteria flourish.

Unfortunately, thoroughly defrosting large items of deep-frozen food requires large amounts of energy and can take a considerable amount of time. In a modern jumbo jet in which food is served to more than 400 passengers, the required amount of energy is not available and time is short, with flights often only a few hours long and passengers waiting to be fed. So it was the airlines which were the driving force behind the introduction of cook-chill foods, soon to be taken up by major supermarket chains.

When the Wakefield Health Authority made public its cook-chill policy, several protests were made by the catering staff, the unions and the medical staff. A meeting was called, at which I expressed my view that to add cook-chill to the already haphazard system in Stanley Royd would produce food that would be not only of low nutritional value but also potentially dangerous. Although my protests had little effect on a majority of members of the health authority, some grew concerned and one of those leaked the minutes of the meeting to the press.

The *Yorkshire Post* broke the story, quoting from the minutes that I had described cook-chill as 'microbiologically unsound and nutritionally unsafe' (although my actual words were 'microbiologically unsafe and nutritionally unsound'). The *Yorkshire Post* story was taken up by the national press and, in particular, by the *Daily Telegraph*. Suddenly an avalanche of criticism fell upon my head, and the first of many serious efforts were made to undermine my standing as a scientist.

For a start, I attracted the fury of two leading members of the Yorkshire health bureaucracy. One was the then Brian Askew, now Sir Brian, chairman of the Yorkshire Regional Health Authority, who was by trade a brewer with a company already committed to serving cook-chill foods in its pubs. The second was Brian Birchall, district general manager at Wakefield Health Authority, who had previously worked for United Biscuits, which also had cook-chill operations. One of Birchall's tasks was to impose some control on the cash-strapped Wakefield Health Authority finances. (He was to die some time later from meningitis.)

This, however, was not merely a provincial row. There is, in London, an organization known as the Food Hygiene Bureau which, although it does not make too much use of the point, is funded by the food industry; it is one of the most powerful pressure groups in the land. In July 1987, it called a meeting at the London Hilton Hotel to dispel fears about cook-chill. A pre-meeting press release, read to me by a reporter at Radio Leeds, accused me of 'putting patients' lives at risk'. At the meeting, a statement was made saying 'Professor Lacey is leaving himself open to the challenge that he has other interests at heart besides the public's.'

These statements were not only insulting but baffling. The first, that I was putting patients' lives at risk, was patently a contradiction of the truth: I made my protest at the health authority meeting. The second, I discovered later, had been drawn from the fact that I had advised another London-based food safety advisory committee, the London Food Commission, a charity largely funded by the then Greater London Council. Although I supported its work, I never accepted a fee. The committee, unlike the Food Hygiene Bureau, was totally independent of the food industry or any other outside interests and that, to me, suggested that any of its findings were untainted.

I felt I had no choice but to sue. I had not, of course, been invited to the Hilton Hotel meeting but the Medical Defence Union solicitors, Hempsons, discovered that the two attacks had originated from a David Edwards and Professor George Glew, of the then Huddersfield Polytechnic Catering Department. Edwards offered an apology and a retraction, which we accepted. Professor Glew was more obdurate and we were eventually forced to issue a writ for libel and slander and ask for an injunction that such remarks would not be repeated. On 22 September 1988, the Food Hygiene Bureau issued a formal apology prepared by my lawyer, Andrew Caldecott. The case against Professor Glew was finally settled out of court in January 1989, with agreed costs and damages to me.

In the meantime, back in Yorkshire the cook-chill controversy continued. First, it was discovered that in installing the new system, in which chilled cooked food was reheated in the old kitchen away from the wards, the Wakefield Health Authority had breached a DHSS guideline which insisted that cook-chill food should be reheated 'at the point of consumption' and served 'immediately'. Worse still, perhaps, for the authority accountants, it had also been discovered that the cook-chill method, rather than saving money, would actually need additional resources, including £350,000 for reheating equipment on the wards.

This ongoing row, reported with relish by the local media, led to a public confrontation between the chairman of the Wakefield Health Authority, Sir Jack Smart, who expressed concerns about the extra funding needed to implement the scheme fully, and Brian Birchall, who had strongly backed the Wakefield scheme and led those in the health authority who were happy to spend more money to 'rescue' the existing investment. Eventually, yet another public enquiry was set up and Sir Jack Smart was later dismissed from his post. Birchall became chairman of the Yorkshire regional catering committee and recommended the installation of cook-chill in all 128 hospitals. Many, however, refused to comply.

Yet another war of words began, which there is neither the space nor the need to go into here. It led to the health authority issuing a statement advising the media and public to disregard my statements 'which in the medical and scientific world have been discredited over the past year'. Just who were these scientists who had allegedly 'discredited' my work I never did find out. My lawyers did, however, fire off another letter to the regional health authority, and no similar allegations were ever made again.

After this unpleasant and professionally frustrating episode I could, I suppose, have withdrawn into my laboratory lair, licked my wounds, and taken a vow of silence. From a career and personal point of view, that would have been the sensible thing to do. I might have done, had not a very nasty little micro-organism indeed, by the scientific name of *Listeria monocytogenes*, appeared in the nation's food.

4

COOL SPECIMEN

The disease listeriosis is named in honour of Joseph, Lord Lister, the English surgeon who in the nineteenth century pioneered the use of the antiseptic phenol with surgery when he realized that most surgical deaths were caused not by the trauma of the operations, brutal though they were at the time, but by infections that attacked the open wounds later. His name stands alongside that of Alexander Fleming in the lexicon of towering British medical achievers, but the bacterium that shares in that name is a particularly unpleasant brute.

It had been known for decades that women who worked with sheep, such as the wives of shepherds or workers in slaughterhouses, were, in isolated cases, particularly prone to illnesses during or after pregnancy. They were likely to lose the baby through miscarriage, give birth to stillborn infants or, perhaps worst of all, give birth to infants who were brain-damaged (although this term was not used until recently: these unfortunate youngsters were known, at best, as Simple Simons or, at worst, as imbeciles). Until this century, however, no one knew the cause of these conditions. It is in fact the bacterium *Listeria monocytogenes*, first isolated in a rabbit as recently as 1926. It was then found in an adult human in 1929 and in a baby in 1936. Fortunately, listeriosis was very rare in humans, compared with diseases like tuberculosis, typhoid, diphtheria and others, which killed people in their thousands, and it was therefore not subject to much medical interest.

This disease was associated not just with sheep but also with other animals, in which it attacks the optic nerve, usually in one eye only. This causes the unfortunate animal to go blind in the infected eye and, as a result, walk round and round in unsteady circles as though drunk. Significantly, although no one noticed this for many years, these conditions usually arose either in late winter or early spring, when the weather was still cold.

For almost 50 years, no one really understood how the disease infected humans. Then in 1981, there was a serious outbreak of listeriosis in eastern Canada. The outbreak attracted public interest for the first time, because of its cost in human terms: of the 41 victims, 34 were pregnant women, and 16 of their babies died either by miscarriage, stillbirth or soon after birth. Of the other seven victims, six contracted meningitis and two of them died.

The tragedy set alarm bells ringing and resulted in a high-level investigation and research project by both Canadian and American doctors and scientists. They soon discovered that all the victims had eaten from the same batch of coleslaw, a mixture of cabbage, radishes and carrots, which had been kept in cool conditions for most of the preceding winter. Before sale, the vegetables had been coated in mayonnaise, and the finished product had been kept refrigerated for several weeks before being sold.

The investigators tracked down the source of the coleslaw and from there tracked the ingredients to a nearby farm. There, they discovered that the cabbages had been grown on a field which had previously been grazed by sheep and had, therefore, been richly fertilized by sheep droppings. This finding began to jog scientists' memories: they remembered that shepherds' wives were prone to miscarriage, and the second key factor, the fact that listeriosis infections in sheep were more likely to occur when the weather is cold. Could there be a link?

The *L. monocytogenes* which had attacked the pregnant women and other victims had been isolated and identified as a particular type known as *4b*. This was submitted to exhaustive tests, and a particularly dangerous characteristic was discovered: unlike most other dangerous micro-organisms (salmonella, for instance, can only grow at temperatures between +12°C and + 42°C), this particular bacterium can multiply, admittedly at a slow rate, at a range of temperatures down almost to freezing point. It will continue to grow quite significantly up to +4°C and then go into rapid multiplication at rates almost equivalent to salmonella all the way up to +40°C.

Here was the breakthrough. The original bacteria had come from sheep dung in the cabbage field. It had continued to multiply on the cabbages during winter storage. Then it was given an enormous boost: the mayonnaise added to the coleslaw was in fact a new source of nutrition for the bacteria, allowing it to go into a new, increased multiplication phase. If any of those victims had allowed it to remain in relative warmth in their kitchens or in bowls on their dining tables, that multiplication rate would have reached astronomical rates.

The true significance of the Canadian outbreak was that the initial stages of this disease's growth took place either in cool storage or under refrigeration. Hitherto the refrigerator, in most ways one of the greatest improvements in food-storage techniques ever invented by human beings, was widely regarded as the ultimate safeguard in ordinary household food hygiene. It still is in some quarters, but now a little-known bug, which had rarely before attacked people in large numbers, had turned that refrigerated environment to its own advantage. The humble fridge, an integral part of the lifestyle of the developed world, a necessity so common as to be as much part of every kitchen as the cooker itself, was no longer a foolproof method of food storage. This should have set alarm bells ringing throughout the world. It didn't. In fact, as far as I can tell, the news never reached Britain – certainly, it never came to my attention and as a leading professional in the field, I would have been one of the first to know. I make it my business, as far as I am able, to keep abreast with the thousands of research findings published throughout the world each year. As far as I know, these had never been published in Britain.

Five years later, the Thatcher Government 'reforms' of the National Health Service were getting into full swing, and, in order to cut costs, many hospital services were being privatized and put out to tender: cleaning, laundry, porterage, even some medical services like pathology. The Stanley Royd outcry had been seized upon by the government as the ideal opportunity for also putting out to tender hospital catering, which accounted for a very large slice indeed of the NHS's multi-billion-pound budget. Following the Wakefield Health Authority's decision to install new cooking technology in its six hospitals, the government had taken to these new methods with enthusiasm and was ordering that it should be installed in something like 1,000 hospitals throughout the country.

The new panacea that would save all this cash was cook-chill, that method of preparing food up to five days before consumption and heating it through immediately before serving. There were many flaws in this programme, not the least being that, instead of saving costs over the coming years, it was to cost an estimated £500 million or more in extra expenditure – £1.5 million in Wakefield alone. It has now been abandoned by many of the health authorities, which had accepted it with reluctance: the reheating required to make cook-chill food safe, as well as being costly, reduces the nutritional value and acceptability of the food. The major flaw, however, the potentially lethal one, was scientific, and it had been either overlooked or ignored. This was that cook-chill food is usually stored at a temperature of between +1°C and +4°C, exactly the temperature range at which the Canadian listeriosis outbreak had begun its fatal course.

Although I was still at this time unaware of the Canadian research, I was aware of – and had expressed during the Wakefield incident – growing doubts on the efficacy of cook-chill as a safe method of storing food. In particular, I had heard that experiments carried out by the Public Health Laboratory Service in Northern Ireland that had shown that cook-chill and subsequent reheating to the then-required temperatures did not kill listeria bacteria. However, public health laboratories were not permitted to publish the findings of such experiments without the permission of the Department of Health in London. In this particular case, permission had not been granted.

One day, one of the staff at my laboratory in Wakefield asked me if I had seen an article about the growth of bacteria at low temperatures in an American technical magazine called the *Journal of Food Protection*. I had not, so he showed me the article, by a Dr Palumbo. This outlined the findings of the Canadian research and other cases, including an outbreak in Los Angeles in which listeria in a soft cheese particularly popular with Mexican immigrants had led to 148 cases and 48 deaths. I read this with alarm, for it came just as it was becoming clear that cook-chill was to be imposed in virtually every hospital in the country.

This was, of course, both medical and political dynamite. I knew that to make a case that would be listened to, I had to have some scientific findings fully researched here in Britain. An article in a somewhat obscure American journal, however responsible, would not stop the NHS cook-chill juggernaut and the powerful politicians who were imposing it. I ordered, as was my right as a research professor and my duty as a public-health civil servant, an immediate investigation of cook-chill safety with particular reference to the ability of listeria to multiply at low temperatures. It would take some time and, regrettably, our most emphatic points were to be made for us by the tragedies that were to befall two young mothers-to-be.

One of the problems in detecting listeria in pregnant women is that, for the woman at least, the symptoms are relatively minor: a short outbreak of flu-like symptoms which pass in a day or so. If the woman does consult her doctor, and I would estimate that this happens in less than one in ten cases, her symptoms tend to be dismissed as either influenza or a minor urinary ailment and treated as such. When the symptoms pass, the incident is soon forgotten. Until, of course, she miscarries or gives birth to either a stillborn child or one with severe brain damage.

The reason for this effect is simple. Usually – and this would happen in the case of a healthy pregnant woman – listeria falls prey fairly easily to the body's natural defence mechanisms, such as cells which track down and kill harmful invaders. Under certain conditions, this does not happen. If, for instance, the victim is taking steroid drugs, has cancer, liver damage or renal disease, or is very elderly, the body's defences have already been weakened and the listeria can cause serious illness or sometimes death. For a baby in the womb, listeria is extremely dangerous because, as I explained earlier, an unborn baby has no immune defences and acquires those only after birth. When the bacteria attacks, it produces large amounts of a toxin called listeriolysin. This invades the unborn baby's brain and causes damage which can either kill in the womb or create serious illness only noticed at birth. The listeriosis can still be treated in the newly born child, so that it survives physically, but the brain damage is, alas, irreversible.

With our research programme underway in Leeds, we were alerted to the case of a 26-year-old woman who already had one healthy child, a daughter, but who gave birth to a stillborn child in 1988, after some days of a flu-like illness. Samples were sent to my laboratory, and we discovered that both mother and baby were infected by *L. monocytogenes*. We made all the attempts we could to establish what the woman had eaten in the ten days before she fell ill but, sadly for our research, her waste bins had been emptied and cleaned, and the contents of her fridge were not affected. We did establish, however, that she was very fond of soft cheeses, both English types and imported varieties like Camembert and Brie.

This raised our suspicions, as soft cheese was known to be a potential breeding ground for listeria, and those suspicions were to be bolstered later on by other outbreaks involving soft cheeses, but suspicion is not scientific proof. That was to come a few weeks later.

The victim was a baby stillborn to a 31-year-old woman after a 24-hour outbreak of a flu-like illness. From samples, we found that both mother and fetus had been affected by *L. monocytogenes* 4. She told us that five days before her illness struck, she had bought a cook-chill chicken from a supermarket and had eaten some of it the same evening. The remains were kept in the refrigerator for three more days and then eaten cold with a salad. We discovered the carcass of the chicken in the woman's dustbin, and lo and behold, we found that the chicken was infected with exactly the same *L. monocytogenes* 4 which had infected the mother and killed the fetus.

This was the concrete proof we had been seeking. So concerned were we to check our findings that we sent off samples of the bacteria to the world-renowned Institut Pasteur in Paris. There, Dr Jocelyne Rocourt conducted an independent examination and came up with identical findings: the bacteria in the mother, the fetus and the chicken remains were from the same source.

With a major scientific discovery on our hands important to the future health of the nation, I and my team of investigators – Dr Kevin Kerr and Dr Stephen Dealler – believed it was greatly in the public interest that such knowledge should be shared as widely as possible. This was particularly so because hospitals were installing cook-chill systems, and because the supermarket chains were selling cook-chill in ever-growing numbers, appealing to working mothers for whom they were a time-saving way of preparing meals – millions of portions were already being sold every year. So, as soon as we were convinced that our findings were proved beyond doubt, we reported them through 'the normal channels' – i.e. they were published in *The Lancet*, which is read by every doctor in Britain and by many thousands more around the world. These readers, I presume, include the medical people in the Department of Health.

We expected immediate action from the Department of Health. Instead, we met obfuscation and delay (for instance, it was not until a year later, in 1989, that the House of Commons Select Committee reported its findings, following which the Department of Health warned pregnant women to avoid eating potentially dangerous food) which, in me at least, brought on an ever-growing feeling of frustration. Then in March 1988, it was revealed that a new hospital was to be built in Halifax without any kitchens at all: its food was to be supplied entirely by outside caterers on the cook-chill system. This decision caused some anxiety in the Pennine mill-town, and I received a call from the *Halifax Courier* asking me if I thought the system was safe. I could, of course, have said 'no comment' but decided that to sit on the truth would make speculation even more confused. I thought it was time that the facts were made public; also, responsible as I was for public health, I believed that it was in the interests of public health that I should put the facts to the public. I said that, in my opinion, the planned cook-chill system could not guarantee to kill listeria.

I was by now not the only voice in the wilderness expressing doubts about cook-chill (I will not name others here, as I do not wish to jeopardize their careers). The *Sunday Times* carried several articles, and the well-respected *New Scientist* magazine carried a piece on cook-chill and listeria in July 1988, in which my views were quoted. However the *New Scientist* also quoted an unnamed spokesman from the Department of Health, accusing me of 'listeria hysteria'.

Professional colleagues began to write letters to *The Lancet* to undermine our findings. One correspondent's view coincided with the official Government attitude that the listeria debate was little more than a storm in a teacup, arguing that only two cases of listeria poisoning had been reported in the United Kingdom. These two were not, as it happened, the two that my colleagues and I had confirmed in Leeds.

My colleagues Drs Kerr, Dealler and I fired off a joint reply to *The Lancet* which was printed on 12 November 1988, outlining our investigations into the two miscarriages we had studied and added:

Outbreaks of listeriosis with case fatality rates of up to 47 per cent have repeatedly emphasised the role of contaminated foodstuffs in the transmission of the disease. Many sporadic cases are probably food related too ... We agree with the recommendation that pregnant women avoid chicken products and other food which may contain *Listeria monocytogenes* unless these foods are known to have been cooked thoroughly by a method that will reliably destroy this organism. Any food that is not consumed immediately should be discarded.

Now it so happens that *The Lancet* is read not only by doctors and scientists but also by the medical correspondents of all the national newspapers. Within hours of the publication of our letter, the telephones began to ring in the Leeds laboratory and listeria became front-page news; television documentary programmes also took up the case.

One of the television teams that came up to Leeds was from Thames Television's documentary programme, *This Week*. After their long interrogation, I persuaded them that one of the key dangers of cook-chill foods in supermarkets was that, even though they were invariably displayed in chiller cabinets which claimed to operate in the +1° to +3°C temperature range, listeria could still multiply in these conditions, albeit at a slow rate. Moreover, in my opinion, these very low temperatures were only sporadically maintained because of the heat of the surrounding air and the radiant heat that the food was subject to from display lighting.

The director asked me if I were prepared to back this theory by doing an experiment with them. Would I go to the same supermarket that had sold the infected chicken to our unfortunate miscarriage victim and take temperature readings of goods on sale? Now this was something of a challenge. To have set up such an experiment officially by enlisting the cooperation of the supermarket would, of course, have been worthless: forewarned, the managers would have ensured that all temperature targets were met.

So I agreed, somewhat reluctantly, to go to the supermarket concerned carrying a highly accurate temperature probe which we proposed to insert into various cook-chill dishes. I was to be accompanied by one of the television crew carrying a concealed camera and a reporter with a concealed tape-recorder.

Modern supermarkets, of course, employ security cameras on constant lookout for shop-lifters or other forms of suspicious behaviour

– such as tampering with foods. Sure enough, someone picked up the puzzling sight of three men huddled round the cook-chill displays, one of them inserting a strange-looking instrument into various foodstuffs. The security men pounced.

In the confusion that followed, the television crew managed to disappear. I was taken to the manager's office, where my temperature probe, which is merely an advanced and very accurate thermometer, was inspected with great caution. When I tried to explain that I was a professor from Leeds University, the manager and security men plainly believed that I was a madman – and where was this television crew that I was talking about?

When I produced identification, they began to believe my story and, if anything, their attitude turned more hostile. It was illegal, they explained, to tamper with food until one had actually purchased it; it was the supermarket's property until it was actually paid for at the checkout tills; you were not even allowed to measure temperatures in the trolley on the way to the checkout. The police must be called because it was company policy to prosecute in all such cases without exception.

Now this I could really do without. I was already being criticized by various government departments (through the media and the food industry's trade magazines), and to be dragged before the magistrates on some charge would only give credence to efforts to discredit me. I therefore decided to fight back. Such a case, I said, would undoubtedly attract public attention, and this was, after all, the very supermarket whose food had caused the miscarriage cited in our investigation, which was still figuring large in the national press. Did the supermarket really want such publicity?

With that, they let me go. Despite the interruption to the test, I had made one important discovery: of those few samples I had tested, all had been above the recommended temperature levels. When the *This Week* programme, reporting this, appeared a few days later, it was to fan the flames of the controversy.

During those last few months of 1988 I became a media figure. I had participated in over 50 television programmes and 100 radio programmes, as well as contributing to or being quoted in countless magazines and newspapers. I was variously portrayed as either a knight in shining armour or an obsessive hysteric, depending on the parties involved. I was, of course, neither: just a scientist and a civil servant doing the job he was paid to do. My actions were, finally, to make a difference in government food policy, but not for a very long time. In the meantime, I had succeeded in making enemies of the Department of Health, some of my professional colleagues, the supermarket chains and the food-processing industry. And, as the listeria saga continued, I was about to add another to the list: the cooking appliance industry.

5

MICROWAVES UNDER THE MICROSCOPE

Readers will by now understand that microbes, some of the smallest living organisms known to science, can have a major effect on the way we human beings live. Or even die. But in the 1980s, as the science of microbiology explored new frontiers, we were only just beginning to understand just how adaptable these tiny creatures – which include viruses, prions, bacteria and other organisms – are, how quick they are to take advantage of new opportunities for expansion into new environments. And as food technology progressed rapidly during that decade, human ingenuity and the profit motive worked together, unwittingly presenting bacteria with whole new worlds to conquer.

Bacteria have been alive on this planet for millions of years, far longer than modern man. With the balance of nature finely tuned, they had remained in a more or less constant state for many centuries. Since those that are harmful to human beings had been largely brought under control by medical science and discoveries like antisepsis and antibiotics, by the 1960s we thought we understood bacteria and had finally brought disease under control. We were wrong.

Listeriosis is a particularly dramatic example of bacterial disease which, for most of humankind's existence, had confined its attacks to sheep, rabbits and a few other mammals, taking as a victim only the occasional shepherd's wife's unborn child, until the Canadian outbreak in 1981, which showed that *Listeria monocytogenes* had escaped the relative confines of the sheep pasture and established a firm foothold in the production chain for human food. Like any colonial invader of a new world, it would not – and probably never will – give up its new possessions without a struggle. We can never send it back to the meadow but we can, or should, learn how to fight it. But, as in many a war, we lost some crucial early battles.

With the ineffectiveness of refrigeration as a protective measure ignored, we plunged ahead with the cook-chill food process, leaving many consumers unaware of the need to prepare this new diet with considerable care. And there was another dangerous or even fatal chink in our armour: the microwave oven. Here, it seemed to the consumer, was another piece of wonder-technology to make life easier for busy people. The trouble was that thousands, perhaps millions, of British families bought microwave ovens under a delusion.

Just how this came about I am not sure but, when the microwave arrived as the brightest new gadget on the block, there was a belief that it cooked from the inside out. I am not accusing the manufacturers of fostering this belief, for I have no evidence of that but, nevertheless, this became popular myth. Implicit in this was the false belief that, because food was heated from the inside, harmful bacteria in the centre of the dish were killed almost instantaneously. (In fact microwave ovens generate heat by molecular agitation on the outside 1–2cm ($^1/_2$–$^3/_4$in) of the food.) This was a very dangerous assumption, particularly when frozen food was being cooked without being thoroughly defrosted: if the centres of large items of frozen food are not defrosted, cooking will burn the outside before the centre is heated to a temperature high enough to destroy potentially dangerous bacteria, including listeria and salmonella, which are quite capable of surviving the freezing process and becoming active and dangerous again unless they are killed by cooking.

However, the halo around the microwave soon began to slip. As early as 1985, important research, again carried out in the United States, showed that many microwave ovens left 'cold spots' inside food they were supposed to have cooked. For most people, the greatest concern about this was that the food, uncooked, would not taste appetizing. Microbiologists, however, knew that this threatened much more serious consequences. In response, microwave manufacturers, riding a worldwide sales boom with this relatively new gadget, began to build revolving turntables into their machines, assuring new customers that this would solve the cold-spot problem by ensuring that all parts of a dish were subject to cooking.

This, in itself, was not a satisfactory response, as rotation did not ensure that the centres of large items were cooked. Unfortunately, it coincided in Britain with another trend, largely inspired by the microwave craze: the huge rise in consumption of frozen and chilled meals made largely from minced meats – often, at the lower end of the market, from parts of an animal carcass which could not have been sold on the ordinary butcher's slab: ears, skull meat, intestines, parts of the hide and even ground bone and gristle.

One does not have too look too far for the commercial motive behind this: profit. Using parts of an animal that had formerly been discarded increased the value of that animal and provided a new source of relatively cheap protein. In a country where foodstuffs like sausages and meat pies were a regular part of the diet, it was possible to sell these cheaper meats in industrial quantities: at the time, no one questioned what went into a sausage or a meat pie. Foreign dishes that had recently found their way into the British diet – burgers from the United States, spaghetti Bolognaise, lasagnes and other pasta accompaniments from Italy – also provided ways of cooking and selling in huge quantities of meats which, otherwise, would have been destroyed.

I hasten to point out that these inferior portions of meat were not in themselves dangerous: offals such as tripe, sheep's head, pig's cheek, chittlings and others had until comparatively recently been a staple part of the working-class diet of this country. Although not particularly appetizing to the eye, they were and are perfectly wholesome – if cooked properly. That usually means oven roasting or casseroling for very long periods of time, long enough to make tough meat edible and also to kill off most infectious bacteria.

Bacteriologists, however, know that the inherent danger in this process is the amount of mincing done in the factory processing of such meat dishes for the frozen or cook-chill markets. However careful the preparation of a piece of meat, it can pick up bacterial infections either in the slaughterhouse or in the food-processing plant, from either its own guts, handling by humans or bacteria lurking in the food plant itself. Although it must be said that hygiene regulations are very strict in all these areas, no one has ever, nor will ever, invent a foolproof system where human error is impossible.

Surface contamination of meat has been with us since human beings began to walk upright. Indeed, during the hanging process, these surface bacteria are in part responsible for tenderizing it, making it easier to chew and improved in flavour. Now mincing meat on an industrial scale breaks up those colonies of bacteria and spreads them evenly throughout the food made out of the mince – often burying them right in the centre of, say, a burger where the least heat will penetrate. By fast-freezing (i.e. lowering the temperature of food from room temperature to about -20°C very rapidly; deep-freezing is the holding of frozen food) or chilling (cooling food and holding it at temperatures just above freezing point), we are carefully wrapping the deadly bacteria in a cocoon where it will lie dormant until someone gives it the opportunity to strike – unless it thaws out in a faulty supermarket display freezer, in which case the bacteria will become active and multiply even sooner. Then, as often or not, we present it to the microwave oven, which is the bacteria's saviour, as I was to prove.

In 1989, my research department at Leeds began to turn its attention to the microwave oven. In particular, we were determined to disprove the myth that such ovens cook from the inside out and were, therefore, powerful weapons in the fight against food poisoning. Even I was surprised by the results.

We bought ten of the most common ovens on the market and set up a series of tests using various types of cook-chill and frozen foods readily available in any supermarket. We found that the heat created by microwaves was mostly concentrated in the outer surfaces of the food, which is totally inadequate for an item likely to contain harmful bacteria, such as a cook-chill chicken. In ready-made meals, often featuring mince as the major ingredient, we also found that the levels of salt used in the recipe had the curious effect of concentrating the microwaves on the surface of the food, causing it to bubble and quickly become overcooked to the point of burning. A home cook who judged only by eye would assume was the dish was thoroughly cooked – indeed virtually overcooked.

In all cases, the temperature of the food's inner core did not reach and maintain the temperature of +70°C for two minutes, which we had established was the minimum exposure needed to kill all dangerous bacteria likely to be in food, including listeria. Much worse was the final conclusion: 22 out of 27 of the cook-chill meals we tested still contained *L. monocytogenes* after they had been cooked exactly to the manufacturer's specifications.

I do not contend that the results of such a small-scale trial, a failure rate of almost 80 per cent, could be extrapolated to a national scale.

However, had only one of the 27 meals still been infected after cooking, if that failure rate of almost four per cent were projected on a national scale, with millions of cook-chill meals being sold in Britain virtually every day, it could represent a health hazard to thousands of people, were listeria to be present in the first place.

All this we discovered whilst the rush to install cook-chill in 1,000 British hospitals was in full swing. Many cook-chill systems, including part of the Wakefield system, use microwave ovens to reheat chilled cooked food.

What to do? Obviously, it was necessary to pass this information on to the Department of Health which, as far as I knew, was still digesting the facts we had presented them about the multiplication of listeria at low temperatures. In this case the government responded positively and ordered a larger-scale microwave research programme at the state-run Bristol Institute for Food Research. But it was to be many months before it produced any results.

By the summer of 1989, the salmonella-in-eggs panic had arrived (which I will describe in chapter six) and, momentarily at least, listeria and the associated problems with microwave ovens were pushed into the background of the public consciousness. But as the holiday season approached, they were to return.

First, though, there was a case concerning another little-known bacterium, *Clostridium botulinum* or, to name the highly virulent disease this causes, botulism. The name comes from the Latin word for the humble sausage, *botulus*. The sausage has, over the years, become a regular haunt of the bacterium because, inside at least, it provides the four conditions which it needs to thrive: warmth, moisture, nutrients to feed on and, unusually, a lack of oxygen. The latter can sometimes occur inside foods such as sausages because of chemical reactions that remove this gas, which is, of course, a prerequisite of most other animal life forms.

C. botulinum is a particularly unpleasant bacterium because it is not only life-threatening to humans but also extremely tough. To survive when conditions are not ideal, it turns into virtually indestructible spores, which lie dormant until conditions are right. If it enters the human body, it attacks the key points where nerves pass instructions to muscles, thus causing paralysis and loss of vision accompanied by extreme vomiting. The toxin *C. botulinum* produces is so powerful that an amount the size of a coffee bean, if distributed evenly, could kill the entire population of Britain.

On 13 June 1989, *Today* newspaper, with the headline 'DEADLY BUG IN YOGURT', reported that ten people in Lancashire were seriously ill in hospital, some of them on life-support machines. In a feature explaining this disease, it quoted me as saying: 'There has not been a death from botulism since 1978 but I am worried that we will see a revival. Botulism is the most dangerous of the [food] poisons.'

Although I was not professionally active in this case, having been much quoted by the media during the salmonella crisis I was frequently telephoned by almost any journalist wishing to have food-poisoning outbreaks explained in simple terms, something which the Department of Health were unwilling to do. They looked upon their duty, I presume, to play down any threats to avoid public hysteria, but they did at least advise no one to eat hazelnut yogurt, as the yogurt eaten by the Lancashire victims had been made with hazelnut purée contaminated with botulism before it was added to the yogurt. Supermarkets immediately cleared the product, which had emanated from Kent, from their shelves. Despite the reticence of his department, the Health Secretary, Mr Kenneth Clarke, a man known for being more open than many of his politician colleagues, admitted: 'It is very serious and could be tragic.'

One of the victims died. Many more would have succumbed but for modern life-support machines, because one of the terrifying results of this poison is paralysis of the heart and lungs. Victims, still conscious, feel their breath fading and their heart slowing but are totally helpless to take any remedial action. I watched progress of this outbreak with concern because once again, food taken from supermarket shelves which were supposed to be chilled (and botulism, being quite susceptible to cold, would not have developed had the food been adequately chilled) had caused a food-poisoning outbreak. If botulism were to become widespread again, as listeria and salmonella already had, we would face a public heath disaster.

By this time the House of Commons Select Committee examining the listeria outbreak had published its conclusions. On 30 June, *Today* led its front page with the headline: '26 BABIES KILLED BY FOOD BUG BLUNDER'; the *Guardian's* headline was even more telling: 'SILENCE OVER LISTERIA "COST BABIES' LIVES"'. The day before, the Select Committee had found that in 1988 at least 26 unborn and newborn babies had lost their lives because the government had failed to warn pregnant women of the dangers of listeria – the very warning I had reported in *The Lancet* the previous year. (I should point out that the figure of 26 dead or stillborn babies was probably ludicrously low: our figures in Leeds projected a more likely national total of between 100 and 150, which may not all have been known to be caused by listeria.) The *Guardian* reported:

> A unanimous report from the Social Services Select Committee concludes that the department of Health first knew of the link between listeria and food at the end of 1987 but failed to issue a public warning about soft-cheese and cook-chill foods until February this year. We believe that pregnant women could have been alerted to possible hazards far sooner.

The tragic implications of this were illustrated by a case described by *Today* in which a London woman lost her baby after eating hot goat's-milk cheese whilst on holiday in France. Mrs Sally Bourne was quoted as accusing health officials of 'killing my baby' and was reported as saying: 'There should be warning signs in every ante-natal clinic in Britain.'

The chairman of the select committee, Frank Field MP, admonished: 'The government as a whole must take responsibility. They must get their act together.'

The findings of the committee confirmed my own view, quoted by both *Today* and the *Guardian*: 'The government deliberately tried to deceive everyone because a public warning would have got in the way of the boom in cook-chill foods and the privatization of catering in the [National] health service.'

There are some serious questions to be pondered here.

People who criticize my work point out that many more people die from smoking cigarettes, drinking excessive amounts of alcohol or in car accidents than from food poisoning. This is, statistically, quite true. But those people have chosen of their own free will to smoke, drink or travel in motor cars. They are, or should be, aware of the dangers. These babies died because their mothers, in all innocence, took part in that most mundane of human activities, usually believed to be safe: they ate a meal. The death of a baby is a tragedy for any family. That any baby should die when the people elected to govern those victims had in their grasp information that might have adverted the tragedy and failed to use it is a national disgrace.

Why the mothers had not been forewarned of the dangers of certain foods must, for me at least, remain a matter of conjecture. Was it, for instance, sheer incompetence? If so, that means that there are civil servants in the Department of Health who are incapable of recognizing a severe threat to public health when scientific evidence is presented to them. They should be sacked immediately. Was it simple tardiness, the inability of the civil service machine to act quickly in an emergency? If so, their procedures should be streamlined and anyone who obstructs them should also be sacked. Or were the civil servants covering up information? Some of them were scientists like myself, who would be in breach of their scientific consciences to cover up such important public health information. But what would they gain by doing so?

Perhaps we should be looking elsewhere: not at the servants but their masters, the politicians. If the government's first duty is to protect its citizens from harm, is it not paramount to protect them from unnecessary illness? And who would gain by the suppression of information about those illnesses? Only, as far as I can see, the various vested interests of the food industry.

These are, of course, speculations. Whatever the truth about why the public had been denied this information, at least Parliament had taken some of our warnings seriously and the government was now being forced into action at last by media probing. However, any positive feelings brought about by this episode were soon to be dispelled.

During the months after my Leeds team had published a letter in *The Lancet* warning that many microwave ovens failed to heat food evenly to the +70°C temperature needed to ensure that bacteria such as listeria, salmonella and campylobacter are killed, our warning had been taken seriously by many responsible bodies, notably the Consumers'

Association, who argued for the identification of procedures that would ensure safety. Other organizations, including some food producers and major supermarkets, had reacted in a more questionable manner, according to an investigation by the *Guardian*, which concluded that some had merely taken the microwave cooking instructions off cook-chill food packaging rather than replacing them with warnings about the shortcomings of this type of heating. This meant that many thousands of consumers continued to use microwaves without any advice whatsoever. John Beishon, director of the Consumers' Association, would accuse these food producers of a "cover-up". He told the *Guardian*: 'They were well aware of the problems but failed in their obvious duty to alert the public of the dangers.'

The actions of the supermarket chains concerned were indefensible. Now some of the biggest companies in Britain, counting their turnover in billions and their profits in hundreds of millions, they had transformed the way the British people shopped and ate. Yet faced with the possibility that they may in fact be poisoning some of their customers, their first action was to make a difficult situation virtually impossible by removing what little advice on microwave cooking was available. Was this a calculated move taken on commercial grounds, because removing cook-chill products from the shelves would have proved enormously expensive, or was it simply panic? Whatever the answer, fortunately the supermarkets did eventually learn a lesson here: nowadays, when public health is at risk, supermarkets clear suspect items from their shelves almost at the speed of light.

The government's reaction had been considerably slower. Despite the vow of John Gummer, Junior Minister of Agriculture, to look into the matter of food safety with great urgency, it was not until 22 August that he decided to launch a full government investigation into the safety of microwave ovens. The *Daily Express* reported,

A warning went out to Britain's 10 million microwave owners last night after a major inquiry was ordered into the ovens' involvement in food-poisoning scares … Agriculture Minister John Gummer said more than 100 different models would be tested and talks held with food manufacturers about changing cooking instructions on packets.

How many people had become ill from improperly cooked microwave meals in the eight months before the enquiry was launched must be a matter of conjecture. As few as one in ten people approach their GPs with stomach upsets, so only the more serious cases come to light, but an estimate based on our Leeds findings would put the figure into thousands. In view of the earlier condemnation by the House of Commons Select Committee of the listeria 'cover-up' which had cost many babies' lives, the delay was totally unacceptable. Moreover, it suggested that the Ministry of Agriculture, Fisheries and Food (MAFF) and the Department of Health were incapable of any form of emergency measures, however serious the threat.

Just two days after the microwave inquiry was announced, another food hazard hit the headlines. As the *Daily Mirror* put it: 'NEW PERIL IN PATÉ REVEALED BY DOCS: One in 10 samples riddled with bugs.' Stung no doubt by the previous storms of criticism, the government allowed its Chief Medical Officer, Sir Donald Acheson, to reveal that tests had shown that listeria was present in ten per cent of cook-chill pâté samples (as opposed to canned pâté, which is sterile) taken throughout England and Wales.

This particular inquiry had been, by government standards, carried out very quickly for in July, Acheson had issued a warning that pregnant women should avoid cook-chill pâtés – something we had been advocating for a year. Now, despite the results of the new research, which had involved the microbiological examination of 1,774 samples, Acheson saw no reason to expand this advice beyond expectant mothers and other groups whose resistance may have been lowered by age or illness – 'the rest of us can continue to eat the wide variety of pâtés that are now available in shops and delicatessens'.

Here was another case of serious infection of cook-chill foods kept on supermarket chiller shelves which, self-evidently, were not up to necessary standards. I told the *Guardian*: 'This is conclusive proof that that the cook-chill method is inherently unsafe. All pâtés made this way should be withdrawn.' The *Mirror* quoted me: 'We found that 10 per cent of pâté was riddled with listeria over a year ago. I don't know if any deaths have been caused but certainly many people will have fallen ill from it. I can't understand why they have taken this long to issue a warning.'

The Consumers' Association and other groups demanded the setting up of a food safety agency independent of MAFF, which had strong links with the farmers and supermarket retailers. Although this proposal did not come to fruition until almost ten years later (albeit in a watered down version) Sir Donald Acheson's announcement that a new code of practice was to be drawn up with the food industry to control the listeria menace was welcome news.

But what incensed me was that Sir Donald Acheson, the most senior medical adviser in the land, was telling the general public, with certain exceptions, that they could carry on eating food with a 10 per cent chance of it being poisonous. He also pointed out that many of the healthy population already carried small amounts of listeria bacteria in their bodies without ill-effect which, sadly, is also true now that this once comparatively rare micro-organism has colonized the human food chain. But to suggest that we should voluntarily ingest more and increase the risk of food poisoning by eating a non-essential luxury food item was to me inexplicable.

There was only one group which would benefit from continued pâté consumption in those days before proper controls were introduced: the people who manufacture and sell those products.

In December 1989, the results of the microwave research at the Bristol Institute for Food Research were finally announced. They revealed that of 102 models tested, 32 failed to reach the +70°C temperature required to kill dangerous bacteria. Of those, 12 could not even generate +60°C. In other words, if the *Daily Express*'s estimate of there being 10 million microwaves in use in Britain were correct, some 3 million families had potentially dangerous appliances in their kitchens, a population the size of Greater Manchester.

When I first heard these results, I felt that the work of my Leeds University team had been vindicated, and that at last the British public were to be given the public health information to which they were entitled. My pleasure was short-lived, for I was astonished to learn that the names of the appliances which had so badly failed the tests were not to be revealed. The reason for this, said MAFF, was commercial secrecy.

In the public outcry which quite rightly followed it was claimed in some sections of the media that the 102 ovens tested had been *loaned* to the Bristol Institute of Food Research on the understanding that any findings would not be made public. As the institute is government owned, and as the Treasury was imposing swingeing cuts of all government departments, this arrangement presumably saved the taxpayers something like £300,000, a minuscule sum when compared to the size of the department's total budget and surely worth spending on an issue vital to the nation's health.

'Government attempts to alert the public to dangers in microwave ovens have created more heat than light,' retorted the *Daily Telegraph*, normally one of the Tories' most consistent supporters. The *Guardian* demanded: 'If Her Majesty's Government cannot break its pledge of confidentiality, the tests should be re-run on Consumer Association lines: with immediate publication. [The association buys all its test subjects anonymously.] The public eats, so the public has a right to know.'

The government remained silent in the face of such claims. Just as in the case of the listeria cover-up, one can only speculate on their reasons for wishing to keep such information from 10 million anxious microwave users.

In the end, what appeared to be an impasse was broken voluntarily by an organisation known as the AMDEA, the body which represents the microwave manufacturers. Alarmed no doubt by the effect on sales this state of public alarm and confusion might cause, they issued a list of the ovens which had passed the government tests and also a detailed (and, to my mind, confusing) list of cooking instructions for those appliances which had fared more badly. Almost a decade later, I still recommend the use of microwaves ovens only in certain circumstances and with great care (I will give more detailed advice in chapter 17).

In some ways, it was a victory. My Leeds team had succeeded in bringing to the public's attention two major dangers to their health in cook-chill foods and microwave ovens. We had forced the truth into the open, despite the lack of cooperation, to say the least, by the very government departments whose job it was to protect that health, the very people who were employing me and my researchers to do this work.

But it was not the only cover-up on our hands.

6

THE LADY VANISHES

Towards the end of 1986, in the baking heat of Australia, a welcome gust of wind rustled through the hot, humid and malodorous rooms of a slaughterhouse near Brisbane. Welcome, that is, to the people who worked there. For scores of people on the other side of the world, that breeze was to bring distress and pain.

As the gust passed out of an open window, it blew dust from the window ledge into an adjoining field where a crop of mung beans was reaching fruition. The crop involved was not the shoots of the plant but the seeds they had just set. These seeds, sold in their billions in health-food shops and vegetarian stores throughout the world, had since the 1960s become something of a food fad because they are an easily grown, fresh source of protein. Left in warm, dark and damp surroundings, they sprout in a couple of days and need only a minute or so of stir-frying to produce a tasty, crunchy ingredient which is the staple of many Chinese and other Oriental dishes. At home, people grow them in a covered dish; to satisfy the huge demand from the Chinese restaurant industry, commercial suppliers grow them on in propagators made from dustbins.

The seed crop from the Australian field was duly exported to Britain and many of them found their way onto the menus of Chinese restaurants. A few months later, a young mother to be, Kim Webb from Stockport in Cheshire, was taken out for a Chinese meal by her husband, Kevin. This was a celebration, for Kim was no ordinary expectant mother: she was, in fact, carrying triplets which is demanding in the extreme, and was due to go into hospital the following day to complete her pregnancy under medical supervision. The meal was intended as relaxation, a night out to take Kim's mind off her condition, for, should the triplets go to their normal term, there were still some two months to go before they were due.

The following day, Mrs Webb went into hospital but that evening she was stricken with intense abdominal pains. Three days later, the triplets,

29 weeks into the pregnancy, were born. Adam died after just 11 days, despite intensive medical care. Jack died the following day. The third, Ashley, now 11, was later diagnosed to have cerebral palsy. He has spent most of his young life in a wheelchair.

Now, I cannot prove this beyond all doubt, because I did not have the resources necessary to do so, but I strongly suspect that the cause of this tragedy was that mung bean field in Australia. At the time of Kim Webb's troubles, there had been a series of food-poisoning outbreaks in Britain associated with Chinese food, many of which were tracked back (in findings published by the Public Health Laboratory Service in 1987) to the Australian mung-bean crop. There, microbiologists and other health professionals investigated and, in dust samples taken from the abattoir window sills, they discovered several dangerous strains of salmonella. One of them was a type known as *Salmonella heidelburg*, named after German university town where it was first identified.

The various strains of salmonella are responsible for some 40 per cent of all reported food-poisoning cases in Britain. That annual figure for food-poisoning cases passed the 100,000 mark for the first time in 1997. Since estimates suggest that only one in ten people consult their doctor when suffering from a 'stomach bug', we may estimate that approximately one million people are suffering food poisoning each year and that of those some 400,000 are the victims of salmonella. Even these figures are debatable. Although in 1988, *The Lancet* plumped for the ten per cent figure, writing in the *Sunday Times* in the same year, Dr Bernard Rowe estimated that the number of victims who contact their doctors is as low as one in a hundred. If Dr Rowe were correct, the number of total cases of salmonella in Britain would be *four million*. Apart from the treatment costs to those who actually seek medical advice, the costs to the nation in lost working days must be astronomical – not to mention the suffering, which is enormous, especially in the cases of the old, the very young and the already sick.

Perversely, salmonella could, and should be, one of the easiest of the food-poisoning bugs to destroy. It does not naturally breed in the human body: in fact, a healthy human being should not have a single salmonella bacterium in his or her system. Although *S. enteritidis* can survive deep-freezing, it needs relatively high temperatures to multiply fast enough to cause serious illness. It is highly susceptible to the heat of normal cooking: as I pointed out earlier, two minutes at temperatures in excess of +70°C will destroy all salmonella present. It thrives inside the moist and warm conditions found in the guts of most mammals, reptiles and, best of all, birds: the normal blood temperature in birds is 3°C degrees higher than in humans, a perfect environment for its continued propagation.

S. enteritidis is, however, a survivor and will, given the opportunity, become a rampant colonizer of new territories. It would not normally survive in household dust, but it did in the conditions in that Australian abattoir, which were hot and humid. When the bacterium was liberated by that gust of wind, the outside weather was warm, and the mung plants on which it settled would have provided enough moisture for its survival. Those seeds must have been transported in humid conditions and then left to sprout in warm, enclosed and above all damp conditions in propagators of Chinese restaurants, which presented a bacterial paradise, a forcing ground not just for bean sprouts but for their lethal lodgers too. All this could have been negated from a health point of view by proper cooking, but in Chinese restaurants this did not necessarily take place because they were likely to have used another cooking fashion: stir-frying. The theory of this is, of course, that food is cooked over high heat for very short periods of time: two minutes or even less. With a fragile vegetable like a bean sprout, which quickly loses its crispness, this cooking time is often reduced to only a few seconds.

When the Webb family successfully sued for damages (which I will discuss in greater detail in chapter eight) I was to be called in as a key witness because, by that time, I had become embroiled in another food controversy concerning salmonella. The culprit was *S. enteritidis 4*. This time, its source was much closer to home.

During 1984 and 1985, with my colleagues in Leeds, I had been watching with growing concern a puzzling upsurge in the number of food-poisoning cases that were being brought to the notice of our laboratory, a growth of some seven per cent a year (and one which, incidentally, is still going on in 1998: such cases have increased fourfold in the past 12 years). Our analyses showed that by far the largest number of these cases were due to *S. enteritidis 4*.

We were well aware of the fact that this particular salmonella strain lives with great success in birds, with their higher blood temperature.

We knew that *S. enteritidis* lives with its host without causing the host harm, unlike other strains of salmonella which cause illness in the host bird; *S. typhimurium*, for example, is so named because it causes a typhoid-like illness in laboratory mice.

Having noted this rise in food poisoning, our suspicions fell on poultry and, in particular, on battery hens (which produced 95 per cent of the eggs consumed by the public), which are kept in what I believe to be unspeakable conditions in modern factory farms. We postulated that the food poisoning was coming from infected poultry eaten as meat, as the cases were mostly associated with chickens and only rarely with ducks and turkeys. But when we cross-checked our results, the figures did not add up: we found that although the consumption of chicken meat was rising by about two per cent a year, the rise in cases of illness caused by *S. enteritidis* was exceeding that by five per cent. We therefore turned our attention to the only other likely source: eggs.

This glimmering of an idea was by no means as obvious as it may sound. Many people of my age will remember, in our youth, breaking open the occasional 'bad egg' with its breath-catching sulphurous smell. Although a regular source of suspicion and school-boy jokes, this was in fact a fairly rare phenomenon. Many of those eggs would, in fact, have been infected by *S. enteritidis* that had entered the egg from an external source: the shell may have been slightly cracked on laying, and bacteria from the mother hen or farmyard debris would colonize it through the crack. But my research team, though suspicious of the potential health risks of factory farming, knew that battery hens have been bred to lay one egg a day for 300 days and, caged as they are, there is virtually no opportunity for the eggs to be cracked and contaminated. Once released from the hen's body, the egg rolls straight down a chute onto a conveyor belt where it is whisked away for packaging. The hen never has the opportunity to crack it by, say, standing on it clumsily, and there is no farmyard debris in her wire-bottomed cage to harbour bacteria. In this, it appeared, modern factory-farming technology had made a great step forward towards eliminating the legendary 'bad egg'. It was therefore hard to see how eggs could have contributed to the rise in salmonella poisoning in humans.

However, when we began to study factory-farming methods, we discovered facts that were not only morally very disturbing but also potentially lethal from a public health point of view. For, in the race towards fatter profits, battery hens had been turned into cannibals. And as often as not, they were being fed with their own young.

As soon as an unfortunate chick hatches from an egg it is sexed; if found to be a cock – around half the tens of millions of chicks hatched in British factory farms every year – it is taken away to be gassed. Those little corpses were ground up and added to the farm's feed stock. Then they were fed back to the laying hens, so mothers were, in effect, being forced to eat their own offspring. The life of a battery hen is short and brutal: having laid her allotted 300 eggs in 300 days, she too is immediately slaughtered and replaced in her wire prison by a new victim. The hen's carcass is used for many purposes, including being processed into pet food, but on some occasions she was fed to hens in the same battery who were still laying. If any of her eggs have been chosen for breeding and have borne female chicks, this means the hen's carcass could be fed to her own offspring.

Personally, I find this process utterly abhorrent. For man to use his technical superiority to submit other living creatures to such barbarism is objectionable in the extreme. To do so for no other motive than extra profit is morally indefensible.

As a scientist, however, this realization had an even greater impact than moral outrage. For in this discovery we found the answer to our question. *S. enteritidis* was getting into the British egg supply in ever-growing quantities. It was entering the egg not externally through a cracked shell, but internally, from the food the laying hen was being fed. In other words, the bacteria was being built into the egg as it formed in the hen's body, something which to my knowledge had never happened before in the centuries-old relationship between man and domesticated poultry. Man had created a perfect lifecycle for *S. enteritidis*, in which it could go on reproducing itself time and time again whenever a captive hen ate the infected remains of a contaminated chick or hen. The only exit from this continuous cycle was in the infected eggs which went to market – to join the human food chain!

Realizing the significance of our findings, my Leeds team and I began the careful preparation of a scientific paper about the transmission of *S. enteritidis* internally in eggs, which was to be published in the *British*

Food Journal, one of the world's leading food hygiene publications – the normal and proper channel for making known a matter of considerable public concern.

While we did this, I gathered that a series of top-secret meetings had been underway between 1985 and 1988 in Whitehall, for I was not alone in these discoveries. During these three years, the Public Health Laboratory Service in England and Wales had also been plotting the seven per cent annual rise in *S. enteritidis* 4 outbreaks. But, as I said earlier, the scientists who run such labs are not permitted to publish their results in the better-known medical media like *The Lancet* or the *British Food Journal* without permission from the Department of Health. Instead, their figures were contained in their annual reports, literature circulated only to a small number of professionals like myself. Their findings, therefore, were not widely available. The meetings involved officials from the Department of Health and MAFF and commercial representatives from the egg and broiler-chicken industries. The results of the government laboratory tests, although not made known to the general public, had finally wakened civil servants and their political masters to the growing *S. enteritidis* problem and the fact that a major crisis was in the making. For three years, these meetings had agonized over possible solutions.

The agendas of, and decisions taken at, those meetings are still state secrets but, from snippets of information picked up from interested parties over the past decade, I understand that they developed into a straight split between the egg producers and the Department of Health, with MAFF tending to support the producers. Health officials were keen to issue a general warning to the public about how to cook eggs properly and avoid *S. enteritidis* poisoning, a possibility received with open horror by the producers and some of their MAFF allies. In the end, a compromise was reached.

A warning was issued that eggs should be cooked thoroughly at high temperatures so that both yolk and white were hard, but it was issued only to hospitals where patients were already at risk through illness. At the Department of Health, civil servants had managed to cover their own backs by being able to point at a decision which did something to protect the most vulnerable section of the public. But the decision did absolutely nothing for the huge majority of the population, who were *not* in hospital. This would have undoubtedly included several million people who were also at risk: old-age pensioners, to whom eggs are a cheap and easy-to-prepare food; pregnant women and young babies; people already ill from other diseases like kidney problems and non-lethal cancers, or taking drugs like steroids, which would greatly reduce their resistance to *S. enteritidis*.

In other words, the Department of Health failed to carry out its appointed duty to protect the public health of millions of Her Majesty's subjects. How many people died, had their long-term health irreparably damaged, lost their unborn children or became ill in that time is impossible to calculate. But a scientific estimate, based on our Leeds research extrapolated to cover the entire United Kingdom, would run into the hundreds, each case preventable.

And what were the grounds for restricting the public warning only to health professionals in the NHS? The hope of keeping this important truth from the general public so that the interests of the egg producers and their MAFF allies would not be damaged.

The cover-up machine was once more trundling around the land, hoping that doctors and other hospital workers would keep this advice confidential to the management of patients within the NHS. Not only was that an unforgivable breach of public duty, it was also wishful thinking. The NHS, the biggest employer in Europe, has a staff of some half a million people, most of whom put their duty of protecting the public health above that of protecting the reputations of politicians and their civil servants. Inevitably – and not, I hasten to add, from me – the story leaked.

In November 1988, the phone rang in my Leeds laboratory. By then we were already well into our research programme. On the line was a producer from BBC television's consumer programme, *Watchdog*. 'Do you know about these stories circulating about salmonella in eggs?' asked the voice. 'And if so, would you be prepared to come on our programme and talk about the problem?'

I knew that to make public to a huge television audience the facts we had been laboriously gathering for three years would be to cause a major sensation. I also knew that, as two-thirds of my department's expenses at Leeds University were funded by the NHS, in creating such a sensation I was in danger of upsetting the mandarins and politicians who run that service. But I was angry on two counts: at the government's delay in taking action on a serious public-health problem, and at its attempts to cover up a potentially grave situation – by not warning the public at large of the risk of salmonella in eggs, an omission which I assume was to protect commercial interests. 'I'll do it,' I said.

So on that Monday evening in November, along with Dr Tim Lang of the London Food Commission – another food scientist and now a professor at the University of Thames Valley – I went before the cameras and spelled out my fears about *S. enteritidis* in eggs. Our researches had shown, I said, that the disease was endemic in a large majority of British battery-chicken farms. All eggs, including free-range (which come from the same stock as battery hens and are therefore contaminated in their internal organs before they are allocated to either type of husbandry), should be treated with caution. My advice was that all eggs should be cooked until hard. In particular, I advised against the use of raw eggs in the preparation of foods like mayonnaise (my advice on these matters will be given in more detail in chapter 16). Tim Lang backed my findings.

As I was beginning to discover often happens in these situations, the politicians ran for cover. Although the newspapers also took up the hunt, no one in government was prepared to discuss our findings. Until, that Saturday, ITN tracked down the Junior Health Minister, Mrs Edwina Currie, to her constituency in South Derbyshire.

Now, at this time, I had never met Mrs Currie. She was already well known for her outspokenness (and her eagerness to appear on television even in non-political shows) and as I sat watching her on ITN News that Saturday night, I was stunned. For, eschewing the long-winded but quite empty explanations so beloved by other politicians, she told the truth. Asked if the majority of the British egg-laying poultry flock really was contaminated by salmonella, she replied simply: 'Yes.'

Not only was a major politician telling the simple, unvarnished truth: by implication, she was also admitting that both her own ministry, MAFF and other departments had colluded in covering up the scandal for several years. The storm became a hurricane. Much of the noise came from Mrs Currie's Conservative colleagues, many of them backbenchers with rural constituencies, who were clearly infuriated that some of their egg-producing constituents' interests might be harmed by that outrageous commodity, the *truth*!

Watching that news bulletin, I found it difficult to separate my feelings between jubilation and sympathy for this politician. As a lone voice who had been crying in the wilderness for so long on issues of public health, of course I found it greatly satisfying to have my work vindicated in public at this level. But I knew instinctively that Edwina Currie had just committed an act which, although brave, was foolhardy in the extreme from a career perspective.

Her admission was, of course, a huge political gift for the Labour opposition and for the media. With many of her Conservative colleagues against her – I am told that Mrs Thatcher's wrath was awesome to behold – Edwina Currie was 'for the chop'. It did not take long for the axe to fall.

The following month, she was duly summoned to appear before the House of Commons Select Committee on Agriculture. The committee was in itself significant and ominous, because the House also has a Select Committee on Health which, any normal, thinking person would assume, would take prime responsibility when it came to investigating a matter of public health. And since the agricultural committee was stuffed by MAFF and farming-interest supporters in the shape of MPs elected by rural constituents, it was patently obvious that this was not going to be an independent enquiry.

This, presumably, was how Mrs Currie judged the situation, for at first she refused to attend. In the meantime, the farmers and the egg producers were howling for her blood. The singular characteristics of *S. enteritidis* 4 caused widespread confusion: egg producers refused at first to believe that their flocks were infected, because this particular strain can live and thrive within a hen's body without causing the host any harm. The birds were healthy and thriving (if such words could be used under the circumstances in which these unfortunate creatures subsist), ergo, they argued, there was no danger to human health.

Though the scientific advisers working for MAFF and the industry knew this to be nonsense, it was a useful smoke screen to disguise the fact that much of the producers' real anger was directed, not at the scientific facts, but at Mrs Currie's admission that here was a major health problem. If that was so, it may be inferred that some producers, although perhaps not all, were happy to go on knowingly selling contaminated produce so long as the general public was unaware of this fact. In other words, business was more important than the public health.

Following a month of much discussion in the media and charge and counter-charge being bandied across the floor of the House of Commons, and with many of her own party against her, Mrs Currie reluctantly agreed to go before the agricultural select committee. It was obvious that she did not stand a chance of survival without a proper briefing, and I had grave doubts whether her advisers at the Department of Health would provide such a brief. So I wrote her a brief which was both scientifically accurate and, I hoped, clear.

I was wasting my time. Mrs Currie announced her resignation within a few days. The egg producers reacted with a show of self-satisfaction which I found shocking. They seemed to think they had won a great victory. It seemed that the key point evaded them, or they were choosing to ignore it: a junior minister might have resigned, but eggs still contained salmonella.

The government began to act with what I believe was panic – the phrase 'headless chicken' comes irresistibly to mind – in the weeks, months and years that followed the resignation. It announced a number of expensive measures, which, given the lack of control of the breeding flock, must have been expected to have been ineffective. Hundreds of vets were dispatched into the countryside to take samples and conduct tests. Entire flocks found to be heavily infected were slaughtered in their hundreds, and millions of pounds were paid out in compensation to the producers. All this hustle and bustle, which went on for almost three years, seemed to persuade consumers that the government had come to grips with the problem and was finally, if belatedly, trying to protect their interests. This, of course, was the public perception that the government, having suffered a major dent in its image, wanted to create. The trouble was that, although these measures cost tens of millions of pounds, they did virtually nothing at all to eliminate salmonella from the nation's egg production.

As I and other experts had warned, *S. enteritidis* was so endemic that the only way to stamp it out in British egg-laying flocks was to slaughter every hen in the land and start again with completely new stock, a project that would be unsustainable to the public purse. Such an action is probably an impossibility, anyway, because nowhere in the world are there enough breeding hens free of *S. enteritidis* to be the seed corn of such a gigantic operation.

What happened instead was expensive 'patch-and-mend' operation which, in fact, did neither. For the flocks that were slaughtered were replaced with new stock which was already infected. Much of it came from French eggs, and the salmonella problem in France is, if anything, worse than it is here in Britain. In other words, the slaughter policy was a total waste of huge amounts of time and public money.

There was one simple way in which the government could have made a significant advance in reducing, if not eliminating, *S. enteritidis* in our eggs: by banning the feeding of dead male chicks and slaughtered mature females to the remaining flocks. This would have brought to an end the continuous cycle of a new generation being infected from the carcasses of the past one, a cycle that is still permitted more than a decade after the Currie debacle. And why did the government not take such a simple step? I can only assume that by cutting out this 'free' source of protein, egg producers would have to buy in more feed from outside. And that would put up the price of eggs, a possibility that would shock poultry farmers, the huge supermarket chains and the consumer-voter. So our poultry has continued to be extensively contaminated with salmonella, which is why there are so many cases of salmonella poisoning – with the effects I described earlier. But, at long last, there is some good news. The egg industry has recently admitted to me that there is a salmonella problem, and the cannibalism is effectively banned.

That is not a lot to show for ten years work and the loss of a junior minister whose political career now lay in tatters. My efforts also had a personal cost to me and my family, for during this period we began to receive death threats against me, usually telephoned to our home and taken either by my wife or children. We changed telephone numbers and went ex-directory, and the threats stopped. All this came about because Edwina Currie and I told the truth about the poison on our plates. Despite the results, though, I continued to believe it was right, and my duty, to strive to give people a healthier, safer life.

7

LONG-TERM KILLER

In 1982, two very large outbreaks of food poisoning occurred in the United States. Many hundreds of people were struck down with severe abdominal pains and, within days, some 20 people had died. Public health officials quickly traced the outbreaks to burgers provided by two well-known burger chains, which came as a major shock to a country that had made fast food a substantial part of the national diet, in which the burger is king (more than ten per cent of all food spending in the United States goes on take-away meals).

I imagine that the microbiologists investigating the outbreaks were looking for the usual culprits, like salmonella or staphylococci, possibly in the mayonnaise in the salads that Americans habitually eat with their burgers. Instead, they found that another lethal bacterium was increasingly contaminating the human food chain, a complex organism known as *Escherichia coli 0157*, so named for the German Dr Escherich who first isolated this very large family of bacteria in 1886. Poisoning by *E. coli* could cause sudden death amongst its victims, sometimes within five days of the consumption of contaminated food, as in the American outbreak, but few doctors knew at the time that this bug can go on doing its lethal business for up to 30 years after the first infection: 30 per cent of victims, including the majority who recover from the initial illness, subsequently develop renal failure.

The surprise associated with these first two reported outbreaks – which does not mean, of course, that they were the first-ever outbreaks – was that there are many hundreds of strains of *E. coli* that thrive in apparent symbiosis with most living creatures – human beings and other mammals, in particular cattle, birds, even insects – in whom they are either benign, doing no damage at all, or extremely beneficial.

One of the functions of *E. coli* in the gut is to use up any of the excess oxygen that all feeding creatures swallow with their food. This allows other strains of valuable micro-organisms that cannot live in the presence of oxygen, known as *Bacteroides fragilis*, to thrive. These perform two vitally important functions in the healthy body. Firstly, by their very numbers, they prevent other dangerous micro-organisms taking hold: there just aren't the nutrients available. Secondly, they can also synthesize nutrients and vitamins to the benefit of the host animal. One gram of gut material in a healthy human is likely to contain 100 million *E. coli* and a thousand times as many *B. fragilis*.

So these microscopic creatures are present in nature in their trillions and, although *E. coli* had undoubtedly caused many illnesses in human beings over the centuries, most of these would either have been isolated cases or, in the days of more primitive medical technology, simply dismissed as one of many fatal or seriously debilitating illnesses whose causes were unknown. It was only the burgeoning knowledge brought about by microbiology that raised the chilling spectre of a bug previously thought to be benign that had somehow become life-threatening and was common in the human food chain. Why?

In fact, unknown to scientists, the 1982 outbreaks of *E. coli* poisoning in the United States were not the first. In 1955, doctors in Switzerland had begun tracking a new disease that appeared to affect patients, and particularly young patients, in a clearly defined sequence of symptoms. There was an initial phase, lasting about five days, of extreme abdominal pains, diarrhoea and blood loss. Then came ulcers in the gut, which allowed some form of poison or poisons – not yet identified – to escape from the enclosed and normally highly protected gut regions into the rest of the body, where these toxins circulated in the blood stream. They began to attack the red blood cells, which have the vital task of circulating oxygen through the entire body, and to break up into deposits that caused major problems in the body's protein balance; they also began to attack the kidneys, causing even more serious damage. One of the body's key organs, the kidney is also one of the most sensitive. Kidney damage can be irreparable and can, in turn, lead to other severe medical conditions including anaemia, high blood pressure and even damage to the central nervous system, which can cause somnolence, seizure and, in extreme conditions, coma. For those who had suffered kidney failure, regular dialysis on large and expensive 'artificial kidney' machines became a part of everyday life, entailing lengthy and distressing visits to hospital; it was only later that home-dialysis machines became available, and then only for the lucky few. In some cases, a kidney transplant was the only answer, and donor kidneys are always in short supply. For the patients, however, there were no other options: without functioning kidneys to cleanse the body of many impurities, death was inevitable. The Swiss doctors, unable to trace the cause of this illnesses, named the condition Haemolytic Uraemic Syndrome (HUS).

These first findings were taken up in both Europe and the United States, and various potential causes for HUS, such as drugs, cancers and natural infections from bacteria or viruses, were investigated. All these led to a dead end. Even more seriously, it became apparent that HUS was no passing phenomenon, even though for long periods patients seemed to have become cured. Instead, the initial kidney damage and all its related problems seemed self-perpetuating for many sufferers.

In 1982, scientists in the United States finally tracked down the cause of HUS. It was a poison known as *Verocytotoxin* (VTEC), the same poison produced in the human body when *E. coli 0157* escapes from the gut and invades the bloodstream. So here was a chain reaction which should have alarmed every politician, civil servant and doctor in the Department of Health: *E. coli* passing from abattoir to food processor, from food into the human gut, from gut through ulcers into the bloodstream, with the production of VTEC causing HUS and remorseless attacks on the kidneys and other vital organs.

All this could have been prevented by better hygiene in the abattoir, food-processing plant and retail outlet, and, most of all, by proper cooking in the domestic kitchen. All that was required was a few new food-handling regulations and a public warning.

The American outbreaks were soon narrowed down to a particular virulent *E. coli* known as *0157: H7*. This is found in the guts of cattle and is therefore widespread in abattoirs. In cattle, it is usually harmless. In human beings, it turns into a rogue killer. However, as with other dangerous bacteria, there is no reason at all why this organism should enter the human body whilst still active – given proper cooking. Once again, our tried and trusted formula of a cooking temperature of +70°C for a mere two minutes would kill all present *E. coli 0157*.

It now seems so simple, but back in 1982 these lessons had yet to be learned. The culprit, again, was mincing, the process that has the effect of burying surface contamination on meat right in the centre of the product, where heat is unlikely to penetrate – particularly in the then-common process of frying burgers quickly on an open griddle.

In America, a nation which worships hygiene as a god, the news, following the E. coli outbreak, that such contamination could spread from the carnage of a slaughterhouse to a burger bar, another temple of the fast-food cult, was greeted with alarm. Once the danger had been established, the American government took action. American health authorities issued public warnings that people should not eat burgers that were still pink in the middle, which is about the only warning sign that a normal consumer can detect.

New food laws were introduced to protect consumers who purchased their burgers for home consumption, mainly in deep-frozen form. Producers were ordered to label these burgers in such a way as to leave the cook in no doubt that they must be properly defrosted before cooking and must then be cooked at temperatures high enough to ensure the whole burger, and in particular the inner core, reached that vital +70°C level for at least two minutes. These warnings, and the ensuing publicity in the media, ensured that most cooks exceeded these stated minima: the pink-centred burger had been dealt a fatal blow in the United States.

The burger chains, some of the biggest and most powerful business operations in the country, also reacted at speed. Burger-bar hygiene regulations for storage and food handling were tightened and, at vast expense, new cooking methods introduced whereby burgers tend to be cooked in appliances like toasted-sandwich makers, which press onto the meat and cook it from both sides simultaneously, thus ensuring that the heat penetrates the whole centre of the burger, killing harmful bacteria.

So, on the far side of the Atlantic, public health officials were prepared to take the necessary action to protect the public health. The burger chains were willing to invest capital in new equipment and staff training to protect not only their customers but also, of course, their long-term business interests.

In 1983 there were E. coli 0157 incidents in Britain that were brought to the attention of the Department of Health. The British government reacted by setting up a committee. The committee issued its report in 1985 – a full two years after the British outbreak and three years since the cause of HUS was established. It was also three years since the outbreak of *E. coli* in the United States, which one would expect to have been brought to the attention of the Department of Health, as well as the subsequent American legislation. During that time the number of cases of *E. coli* poisoning was growing.

Why there was this unconscionable delay I cannot say, because the deliberations of the committee were not made public. Had they been discussing the threat of war from some new enemy with as-yet-unknown weapons I could perhaps understand. But the fact that this life-threatening organism was known to be simply beatable makes the delay, in my view, inexcusable.

When the committee finally issued its tardy report, it did recommend that warnings should be placed on labels, as had happened in the United States. This would have cost the state nothing, and the costs to the producers and retailers would have been negligible. But even this timid recommendation was ignored by the government. I can only speculate that, once again, the interests of MAFF, the farmers and the food industry were to be put before those of public health: to take such action would acknowledge a public-health hazard in burgers, which might conceivably harm beef sales.

But there would have been other political reasons for protecting the public health. At London's famous children's hospital at Great Ormond Street, a study of 72 HUS victims between 1969 and 1980 showed that only 70 per cent recovered: the remaining 30 per cent seemed doomed to a lifetime of dialysis. If they were lucky enough to receive a suitable donor kidney – they have to be matched very carefully before this major surgery can succeed – they then face the awful possibility that their new kidney might begin to fail at any minute (sometimes, the working life of a donor kidney can be as short as six months). This is human suffering on a pitiful scale. It is also a vast drain on NHS resources. It is estimated that dialysis for a single patient can cost as much as £5,000 per *week*. Taking into account that the Great Ormond Street patients were all youngsters, this could mean treatment for 30 years or more at a cost of £7.8 million per patient. It would be this much should these patients live a full life-span but, on average, it has been calculated that HUS cuts the average life-span by ten years. For very young victims, that figure is likely to be much higher. I mention these figures because by the time the Great

Ormond Street study was published, Margaret Thatcher had been installed in Downing Street as Prime Minister and in her crusade to cut public spending, for the best part of two decades, NHS budgets were to come under merciless review. One of the better ways of reducing public expenditure in the NHS would have been to take a much stronger approach to preventive medicine: it is far cheaper to stop people getting ill in the first place than to treat them. Given the huge costs of treatments like kidney dialysis or transplants, any measure to reduce one of the causes of kidney damage should have made good financial sense.

The long-term effects of the government's refusal to act to prevent E. *coli* poisoning was a growth in the number of cases tracked by the Public Health Laboratory Service's Communicable Disease Surveillance Centre, as the following chart demonstrates:

Reported outbreaks of VTEC-associated illness in England and Wales:

1982	1
1983	6
1984	9
1985	52
1986	77
1987	96
1988	88
1989	178
1990	332
1991	361
1992	470
1993	379
1994	411
1995	804
1996	660
1997	1,060

The government may have decided to dismiss E. *coli 0157* as a serious danger to public health but in Leeds we decided that it was a threat which needed further investigation. In particular, we were worried about the huge increase that took place in the consumption of home-cooked burgers in the 1980s. The reason for this is straightforward: here was a meal which, deep-frozen, was easy to store and, superficially at least, easy to cook; the answer to a working wife's prayer.

In many ways, the burger, a much inferior source of nourishment, had taken over from the traditional British 'fast food', fish and chips, which is high in both protein and energy and, when cooked in vegetable oils as opposed to animal dripping, is a dish with much to commend it. Fish and chips, particularly if supplemented with salad, provides a remarkably balanced meal, but it also has one added advantage: when cooked in extremely hot fat, it is just about as safe as any food can be from a contamination point of view. Fish naturally contains few bacteria capable of causing human food poisoning (if, of course, it is fresh) and any surface contamination caused by poor storage or handling will die virtually instantly in contact with that oil.

This cannot be said for the burger. Made from beef, that comes from abattoirs where many bacteria will live and thrive unless the most stringent hygiene is scrupulously followed, which is then minced – a process that, as I have observed, buries any harmful bacteria deep in the meat – and deep-frozen (the hazard of which, as I explained earlier, being that it is difficult to cook the centres of deep-frozen items without burning the outside surfaces), the burger, of all the poisons likely to be put on our plates, is by far and away the ideal bacterial host.

My Leeds team began a series of experiments to test the hazards created by the deep-frozen, home-cooked burgers sold by all the major supermarket chains and thousands of corner shops. The enemy we were seeking out this time was *E. coli 0157*, particularly hazardous in burgers because the bacteria is present naturally in all cattle.

This time we did not buy our experimental stock from the supermarkets but made it ourselves, following exactly the recipes used in commercial burgers. As with our microwave oven research, we used the 'challenge-test' method, introducing known *E. coli 0157* bacteria onto the surface of batches of beef purchased from retailers. Then we minced the beef, formed the burgers and deep-froze them. Then, following manufacturers' cooking instructions to the letter, we shallow fried 100 experimental 115g (4oz) burgers – our own version of the famed quarter pounder – in open-topped frying pans, the method used for most burger cooking.

Not one of our hundred samples passed the test. *E. coli 0157* survived in every single sample. Had we consumed any burger containing *E. coli 0157* and so cooked, we would have been putting ourselves at risk of almost immediate distressing illness, potential long-term health risks or, at worst, death within a week or so of consumption. For, like other harmful bacteria, *E. coli 0157* multiplies at enormous rates, doubling its numbers every four hours at temperatures as low as +10°C, as illustrated by this rough guide showing the growth rate of a single bacterium:

Approximate growth rates of a single *E. coli 0157* bacterium at +10°C:

4 hours:	2
8 hours:	4
16 hours:	8
20 hours:	16
24 hours:	32
2 days:	1,000
3 days:	30,000
4 days:	1,000,000
5 days:	30,000,000

We should realize that should food be infected, it is highly unlikely that someone would ingest a single bacterium: they are more likely to consume a much larger number. And this table shows the growth rate at a mere +10°C. In the human body, where conditions are damp and nutrients are plentiful and the temperature is +37°C, the growth rate increases. It is little wonder that the body's natural defences are quickly overcome.

Alongside our homemade burger trials we also ran tests on 60 deep-frozen burgers bought from a range of supermarkets, all of which were national names. Again we followed the manufacturer's cooking instructions to the letter. And once again, we had a 100 per cent failure rate: not one of the burgers acheived the crucial +70°C temperature at its centre that must be sustained for two minutes for *E. coli* to be destroyed.

We passed our results directly to the Department of Health, expecting that they would instigate a much broader-based series of trials: our test samples were too few for a full-scale research project and, with our limited resources, we could take the matter no further. At the very least, we hoped that the government would take action, as had happened in the United States, to force the manufacturers to put adequate labels on burger packaging warning about the imperative need for proper cooking. Nothing happened.

On 17 November 1996, 14 years after American microbiologists had first warned of the dangers of E. *coli 0157* in cooked meats, the old-age-pensioners who were regular worshippers at the parish church in the small town of Wishaw, Lanarkshire, sat down for a pre-Christmas lunch. On the menu was steak pie provided by a local butcher, John Barr and Sons, a highly regarded establishment that had over the years won several prizes for its cooked meats and supplied pies and other cold, cooked meats across a large area of Scotland.

Within days, the medical services in Wishaw were overwhelmed as many of those pensioners began to fall desperately ill. By 11 December, 11 had died in great discomfort and, across a large area of Lanarkshire, more and more people were falling ill. Then another outbreak occurred on Tayside, which killed three people. In total, almost 500 people were struck down and the death toll had reached 21 by early the following year. The deaths were quickly attributed to E. *coli 0157*. In Scotland, there was widespread consternation. The Lanarkshire incident caused more deaths than any other known outbreak of E. *coli* poisoning anywhere in the Western world.

Here was a classic case of a food hazard whose causes and effects had been known to food scientists for many years: the potentially lethal danger of cross-contamination between fresh and cooked meats in the same shop where assistants handle both. Fresh meat may be contaminated in the abattoir, in transit or in storage by careless handling, but the contamination is killed if the meat is properly cooked. Cold, cooked meats like ham and tongue that become contaminated do not receive the benefit of further cooking, and so one of the most important safeguards is automatically omitted from the healthy eating chain. Although these meats have already been cooked, either by the butcher or his suppliers, and should therefore be perfectly sterile, sadly the theory fails to recognize human error.

The first and most obvious error is that a butcher or one of his assistants, having handled raw meat for one customer, serves cold, cooked meat to the next. In a busy shop, this probably happens many times a day, and each time the cooked meat is handled there is the risk of cross-contamination. This is a risk which has been known for many years and, in catering establishments, it is a breach of the food-handling regulations to store cooked and raw meats on the same shelf of a refrigerator.

The problem with cold meats in a shop, however, is exacerbated by the length of time which they may remain on sale in a refrigerated display cabinet. These ideally should operate at a temperature of about +3°C, but at the time of the Lanarkshire incident, +8°C was permitted under the hygiene regulations. Even this is not always maintained, for it is generally accepted that most of these cabinets can vary by up to 2°C either way. Given the fact that the cabinets are regularly opened and closed by assistants taking out and replacing dishes of meat, even this is rarely constant, as warm air from the shop wafts in and out. Virtually all these cabinets are floodlit to make the food look more attractive, which in turn adds radiant heat from the lights. There is also the possibility that a refrigerator may be faulty.

Added to this worrying scenario is the fact that meats put on display on the quiet shopping day of Monday might still be there at the weekend, when they are more likely to be sold. Should the temperature in the cabinet have reached +10°C, which is by no means unlikely, a glance at the chart on page 68 will show the potential danger, had the cold meat been contaminated on the Monday. By Saturday, in its tailor-made propagator, a single bacterium of E. coli 0157 could have bred into millions.

I do not yet know the formal findings of the enquiry into the Lanarkshire outbreak, which continues. But old-age pensioners ingesting E. coli 0157 in such huge numbers would stand very little chance of survival. That the death toll in the outbreak was as high as it was suggests that conditions in the butcher's shop that supplied the pies they ate suffered all or some of these hazards.

When the government was pressed for action from north of the border, there came the first stirrings of action on a problem that had been gathering dust in its pigeon hole since 1982. Professor Hugh

Pennington, a scientist from Aberdeen University, was appointed by the Scottish Office to lead an inquiry into the outbreak. It is interesting that the decision to set up the inquiry was taken by the Scottish Office, rather than the Department of Health in London. Pennington's brief was to report to the Secretary of State for Scotland on 'the circumstances which led to the outbreak and the general lessons to be learned'.

According to *The Lancet*, Pennington eventually advised the Secretary on a list of food-handling improvements that would increase safety 'from the farm to the fork'. These included education and awareness programmes for farm workers, stricter enforcement of hygiene laws in abattoirs, the keeping of raw and cooked meats separate in butchers' shops, and better training for all people handling food, including the general public. These were some of the points that my colleagues and I had been urging on the government, by means of numerous articles, letters and evidence submitted to it, for years (although I would have preferred a blanket ban on shops selling both fresh and cooked meats). It took a major disaster to have them become policy, and only then via a non-Whitehall based department of state.

It would be nice to suggest that the 21 deaths were the end of that disaster but that, sadly, is not true. It is highly likely that some of the other 470 victims infected will die prematurely from kidney failure or associated problems in the next decade or so, caused by *E. coli*, although whether their deaths will be officially attributed to the Wishaw outbreak remains to be seen.

When the outbreak was at its height, I was quoted by the *Daily Telegraph* as saying that the eventual death toll could reach 100. When told of this figure, Professor Pennington described it as 'probably on the high side'. But he added: 'I am sorry to say that it is not something one can rule out. A large number of people are seriously ill.'

Worse still, such an outbreak might have been avoided altogether, but for one of the most staggering examples of government neglect of food safety I had encountered in my career so far.

Quite coincidentally during the Lanarkshire outbreak of 1996, a campaign group had been formed in London under the acronym HUSH: Haemolytic Uraemic Syndrome Help (HUS, readers may remember, was the name given to the disease caused by *E. coli 0157* before the link was established). The purpose of HUSH was to take legal action against the

Department of Health and MAFF for their failure to issue warnings about the dangers of infection from improperly cooked food. The group was representing some 30 *E. coli* victims who had suffered grievously as a result of this failure, and asked me to be one of their scientific advisers.

As a result, I found myself studying a mountain of papers on food-safety regulations in the environmental health department in Leeds. There, in the small print, was a regulation issued by MAFF to butchers and other people who sold cold meats in 1995 under the Food Safety (Temperature Control) Regulations. It had been issued in secret without any form of Parliamentary or scientific debate that I have been able to trace: it was approved in September 1995, when Parliament was not sitting, and was not published in Hansard; there was no public scrutiny, and local authorities were merely informed. Far from tightening up the regulations, it substantially relaxed them: the recommended temperature for cold cabinets displaying cooked meats was raised from the then-recommended +6°C to +8°C. Even worse, no time limit was imposed for the display of cold meats at this new, higher temperature.

Given that most cabinets vary by 2°C either way, the relaxing of the rules would have had the immediate effect of providing *E. coli 0157* with the happy breeding ground demonstrated in the chart on page 68 in thousands of shops in Britain. In NHS hospitals, the rules demand that cold meats must be stored at below +3°C, and then only for a maximum of five days. But bacteria, unfortunately, make no differentiation between frail people living at home or those in hospital, as the Scottish outbreak so tragically demonstrated.

The new regulation had therefore put the health of thousands of British people at risk. Who could possibly have benefited from such a change? I can see only one answer to that: the industry that uses hundreds of thousands of such display cabinets. There could be no conceivable benefit for the ordinary consumer. In other words, once again MAFF appeared to have acted in the interests of the food industry by saving them the electricity needed for colder storage and the technical problems of maintaining the +6°C level in cabinets which are being constantly opened and closed.

I believe the secrecy surrounding this decision can only be put down to political expedience. I was not informed, and neither were any of my colleagues in microbiology and allied sciences. This is, as far as I am aware, the first time that this piece of legislation has ever been made public. Had we been informed, some politician or civil servant must have surmised, we would have kicked up another fuss at a time when the public were becoming more and more concerned at the government's inability to ensure a regular supply of poison-free food. So it was slipped in by the back door.

The regulation took effect one year before 21 people were to die in Scotland and 470 more were to suffer severe illness which, even today, may still be threatening their lives. There is good scientific evidence to suggest that but for the extra 2°C it allowed all that suffering might have been prevented. The regulation is still in force today.

8

SOME VICTORIES

As I write this, I am at the end of my professional career. As I shall explain in more detail later, I was forced to give up my tenure at Leeds University and join the Leeds Hospital Trust. My contract, expiring March 1998, was not to be renewed. During the 1980s and 1990s, I became the *bête noire* of some people in high places in the Department of Health and MAFF, and their allies in the farming and food industries. Attempts were made, as I have said, in many different circles – for instance, in the farming and food industry press – to destroy my reputation as a scientist. My life had been threatened, and my wife and children had been subjected to insults and ridicule. But to the question 'was it all worth it?' the answer, with one important *caveat*, is 'yes'. (That exception is the subject the next section of this book.) That apart, there have been some important victories.

I would never claim that I was solely responsible for these, for there were many other scientists involved and dozens of pressure groups like the Consumers' Association, who took up the cause of safer food once that cause had become a major subject for media debate. Perhaps I can claim, however, that I was one of the catalysts for that debate. The media – newspapers and television – deserve much credit. Together we created a situation where the politicians and their minions were forced to take some action – or at least, *appear* to be taking some action.

As a result of the salmonella outbreak at the Stanley Royd Hospital in Wakefield, NHS catering is now much safer, thanks to the abandonment of many hospital trusts of the 'cook-chill' cooking methods which I had fought against so vociferously. It is now standard practice to cook all eggs served in hospital thoroughly, a lesson which I also hope has been learned by other vulnerable people who cook at home: the old, the ill and mothers preparing eggs for young children or for themselves if they are pregnant. Standard medical advice now is that no baby under the age of 12 months should be given any raw egg products.

In the supermarkets, even the least observant shoppers will have noticed major changes in the way that frozen and cook-chill foods are presented. Instead of being displayed in open chiller trays, they now tend to be behind well-insulated doors and kept at temperatures low enough to remain safe even when those doors are opened and closed.

Listeria cases have dropped by 75 per cent. There were approximately 300 cases in 1988 and 1989, and 60 each year from 1995 to 1997. In antenatal clinics throughout the country, expectant mothers are warned against eating cook-chill chicken, pâtés and soft cheeses, advice that arose directly from our listeria research in Leeds. In this great city, with a population of 750,000, not a single child has been born with brain-damage caused by listeria in the past five years.

As safety has increased in the supermarket, so it has at home, helped by food labelling which, although far from perfect, does at least warn the home cook that there are inherent dangers in undercooked food, particularly frozen or cook-chill food. The manufacturers of convenience meals now understand the need to advise customers that the food should be served piping hot. Microwave ovens have become more powerful, so that more heat penetrates the centres of dishes and therefore destroys more bacteria. The very fact that the vast majority of consumers are aware of the dangers of microwave cooking is in itself a major advance. As far as I can judge by personal observation, the microwave is now looked upon as it always should have been: a useful adjunct to the average kitchen, handy for certain peripheral cooking tasks, but not the major cooking appliance.

Although *E. coli* still remains a major hazard, the shockwaves generated by the Lanarkshire outbreak reverberated right into the heart of the meat-production industry, from farm if not quite to fork as the government tried to imply. Hygiene measures in slaughterhouses are now much more stringently enforced, as are storage and display conditions in butchers' shops. There cannot now be a butcher's boy in the land who does not realize the inherent dangers of alternately handling fresh and cooked meats. Many butchers' shops now have two sets of assistants, each exclusively handling either fresh or cooked meats. Those that cannot afford such staffing levels are constantly aware of the need to use different implements like knives or slicing machines for different meats and clean them between using them. I have watched this myself: try buying cooked ham, raw parma ham and then cooked turkey breast at your local supermarket and you will see the slicer cleaned thoroughly between each purchase, a small but extremely important advance.

Now, every local environmental health department in Britain regularly carries out spot checks at local food stores and restaurants, taking samples at random and sending them off to the local public health laboratory for analysis. This is a measure so obvious that it stuns people to be told that it was rarely done until 1990. Thankfully, most of these spot checks prove negative, but they reinforce the message. A shopkeeper who knows that a local health inspector may call at any minute of any day is reminded that, potentially, they could be putting their customers' health and even lives at risk by slack hygiene of the most basic kind – like washing thoroughly after using the lavatory.

Most butchers – and other food handlers, for that matter – have of course been aware of these risks for many years but at peak shopping times, there must always be a temptation to ignore them to serve an impatient queue. The spot check is now a warning against such forgetfulness. Meeting these standards is a prerequisite to staying in business – quite apart from the fact that to be involved in a food-poisoning outbreak will, almost inevitably, attract major media interest and the effect of that on a business can be nothing less than disastrous.

This is the sharp end of government legislation. Much of it came about as a result of one of the safe-food lobby's greater victories, the passing of the Food Safety Act of 1990. It imposed swingeing penalties – producers who breach the regulations can face fines running into tens of thousands of pounds and, even more seriously, can lose their licences to handle food. Negligent or, worse, reckless disregard for food-handling regulations has now become a serious criminal offence. Although the Conservative government made a great play of introducing this key legislation, it appeared to me that they did so only with the greatest reluctance and after many years of warnings which, by and large, were ignored. This was the first time a British government had introduced stringent laws covering a wide gamut of food preparation and sale.

Major advance though the Food Safety Act was, it still fell well short of the prize that we had been pursuing since 1986: the establishment of a government food standards agency totally independent of MAFF.

I have long been irritated by the fact that MAFF is routinely described by both print and broadcasting journalists as simply 'the Ministry of Agriculture'. Admittedly, the Ministry of Agriculture, Fisheries and Food is an unwieldy title, but there are probably millions of ordinary Britons who do not realize that the two final Fs even exist. It is that final F that is of the greatest significance to the average consumer, yet the fact that Food is the last word of the title seems to me to be symbolic of the priorities of this ministry: agriculture comes first, fisheries second, and food a poor third.

People once described the Church of England as 'The Conservative Party at prayer'. Agriculture may be described with some justification as the 'Conservative Party at work'. For generations, the party's grandees have come mainly from the farming and land-owning classes, and even those who are businessmen or professionals tend to take up agriculture as hobby-farmers (some authors have said that as many as 70 per cent of Conservative MPs have commercial links with the food and farming industry). Others who do not work the land use it for sport and recreation. So MAFF has always been a department of state that fitted very snugly with the ideals of the Conservative party.

This affinity between the Conservatives, when in power, and MAFF has long been the subject of heated debate and attack but, until Britain joined the Common Market in 1973, such attacks could be easily deflected. After World War Two, when a run-down farming industry almost led the country into starvation, farming boomed on fat subsidies and capital-intensive agricultural methods that sent production soaring. This, at the time, was perhaps necessary, as the country needed to grow more of its own food. After we joined the EEC (as the Common Market then became), over-production had become a major problem, with billions of pounds being spent to store food mountains and wine lakes. But MAFF sailed on regardless, encouraging more and more production and persuading farmers to take out even bigger loans for the purchase of new machinery, stock and buildings. Apart from a handful of scientists like myself, and conservation groups alarmed at some of the new farming methods and the ever-growing desecration of the British countryside, no one seemed to care.

Food was a minor player until another social change brought a major player into the game: the growth of the nationwide supermarket chains.

They fitted well into the MAFF nest because their needs coincided with those of the farmers: they, too, wanted cheap produce that could be sold at high profit margins. Within the ministry, Food now became almost as important as the Agriculture because it had important clients: the major food processors and supermarket chains, the fastest growth sector of the British economy of the past 20 years.

In November 1996, I was invited to give the annual George Orwell Lecture at Birkbeck College. To give the Orwell lecture is, as its dedication suggests, a high honour in intellectual circles, and the audience tends to include some of the brightest minds in modern radical politics. My lecture was about politics and science, or rather the triumph of the former over the latter. In honour of the author of *1984*, I entitled the lecture 'The Ministry of Agriculture – The Ministry of Truth'.

In it, I described the attempts made by MAFF to cover up the then growing BSE crisis (which I shall describe in depth in the next section of this book). In likening MAFF to the sinister Ministry of Truth in *1984*, I was making the point that, in real life as in fiction, ministerial overlords seem to consider their key role to be covering up the truth, rather than protecting the public that they supposedly serve. In other words, they reverse the role that they have been created to perform: they protect commercial interest from public need, rather than vice versa.

In its report of that lecture, the *Political Quarterly* used some of my comments as sub-headings, which summarize rather neatly my overall condemnation of MAFF: poor advice, inadequate response; sins of omission, sins of commission; BSE and CJD doublethink.

My attacks were based on my experiences of MAFF over the previous ten years, which I have illustrated, and will continue to illustrate in the next section of this book. I launched them because I saw a compelling need to force the government to put an end to the obvious problem in the ministry's character. This was a viewpoint shared by dozens of scientists, politicians, journalists, and pressure groups. By all means, have a ministry responsible for encouraging the good health of British agriculture: it is a vital industry that employs many people and provides, most of the time, high-quality produce. But to have this self-same ministry in charge of policing the safety of its main clients' products is rather like having a football match with a referee appointed from one of the teams – and, indeed, from the team which is favourite to win. This not only presents the referee with a clash of loyalties but also makes any decision he takes suspect.

This is why, from 1986 onwards, I began pressing for the creation of an independent food watchdog, whose sole interest would be to protect the interests of the consumer. There was widespread support for this campaign across a wide cross section of the thinking population. There was one notable exception: the successive Conservative governments. We had to wait for the Labour election victory in May 1997, to see progress towards this ideal.

On 14 January 1998, Dr Jack Cunningham, the new Minister of Agriculture, announced the creation of the Food Standards Agency (FSA) which, it is said, will control food safety standards from 'plough to plate'. When it goes into operation, it will be independent of MAFF, although it will draw some of its staff from there and from several other Whitehall ministries, mainly the Department of Health. It is to have a very wide remit.

It will enforce food-safety regulations from the farm to the consumer's table, although what happens behind the farm gate will still be largely inspected by MAFF officials; with a research budget of some £25 million a year, it will have the final say in advising ministers on pesticides and veterinary medicines; it will be responsible for licensing all abattoirs and, presumably, have the power to close them down if standards are not met; it will draft legislation on the labelling of food and share with the Department of Health the task of advising the public on how to achieve a balanced and healthy diet.

This was the sort of shopping list I would have written myself for the new agency, with one minor reservation: I would have given the FSA the power to investigate behind the farm gate. Some observers immediately seized upon the fact that this work will continue to be carried out by MAFF personnel as a potential area of conflict. The arrangement will, most certainly, depend on the integrity of the MAFF staff on the FSA. However all the information I have received from contacts in the public-health world encourages me to hope that that the FSA, and not MAFF, will hold the whip hand when it comes to ensuring that public health interests are placed before commercial needs. If this is true, and I earnestly hope that it is, in the FSA at last we have a major breakthrough, a true victory for food-safety campaigners. Why it took so long one can only speculate but, I suggest, that after spending so many years defending food policies which, in the end, were proved to be indefensible, the Conservatives dared not create such an agency themselves. The Conservative Party's cosy relationship with landowners, farmers and food processors might also be part of the equation.

Most people judged the creation of the FSA to be a necessary and prudent piece of legislation, but surprisingly, the FSA came under attack from the day of its announcement. The following day, a spokesman for the Food and Drink Association, the powerful food industry lobby group, described the FSA in *The Times* as a 'food poll tax' which would inevitably push up prices. Most criticism concerned the cost of the agency, estimated at some £100 million a year, much of which would be met from a £100-a-year levy on Britain's 600,000 food outlets – the supermarkets, restaurants, take-aways and corner shops.

It is indeed a great deal of money, but in terms of total government spending in the United Kingdom, it is in fact not a large sum. Earlier, I noted that the lifetime cost of kidney dialysis for one young victim of an *E. coli* outbreak could run to more than £8 million. If the FSA prevents just 12 such cases a year, its cost to the country will have been covered. The medical costs of the victims of the two Scottish *E. coli* outbreaks may run into tens of millions of pounds. And *E. coli* is one of the rarer forms of food poisoning: the costs to the nation of salmonella – with reported cases alone now exceeding 400,000 a year and an estimated four million more going unreported – are incalculable, particularly if one includes the millions of working days lost from 'stomach bugs'. If the FSA can prevent just a small percentage of such outbreaks with a combination of more stringent safety standards and well-presented public advice on safe cooking, it will repay its budget time and time again.

I am playing the politicians' game here, counting the cost of preventable illness in pounds and pence, only to counter those who critize the FSA. What I believe is important is the power it will have to prevent the human cost in pain, grief and suffering of lives unnecessarily shattered by the poisons on our plates.

One example of such suffering is the pain, bewilderment and grief caused to Mrs Kim Webb by a meal in a Chinese restaurant in Hazel Grove, South Manchester, which has still not ended 11 years later. Mrs

Webb, as I mentioned in chapter six, was the lady whose triplets arrived six weeks prematurely.

Only Ashley survived, brain-damaged by cerebral palsy. He spends most of his time in a wheelchair, attended constantly by his mother. His condition means that he is unlikely to reach the age of 50. Kim and Kevin have adopted a daughter to complete their grievously curtailed family, but will never forget the two sons who never had a chance to experience life.

Tests carried out in hospital when Kim first fell ill showed that she was infected with *Salmonella heidelberg*. At first, suspicion fell on a salad she had been given in hospital two hours before she fell ill. The Webbs' deep grief flared into anger at the thought that, having taking every sensible precaution they could imagine, their babies might have died as a result of negligence in the hospital which was supposed to nurture and protect their future family. They took legal advice and sued, but there was a deep flaw in their case: *S. heidelberg* can be and is a killer, particularly to unborn children, but there has never been a recorded case of it acting so lethally within 150 minutes.

The case dragged on for almost five years, but the veracity of the medical evidence was in doubt. In 1991, their lawyers decided they must have an independent second opinion and asked me if I would look at the case. I did so with great interest, for I too was puzzled at the speed with which this outbreak had seemingly occurred. It was only after going through the medical notes, and seeing Mrs Webb at her home, that I learned about the Chinese meal eaten almost exactly 24 hours before she was taken ill.

This is precisely the time span one would expect between a heavily pregnant woman ingesting *S. heidelberg* and becoming ill. Having made this point to the lawyers, the case against the hospital authorities was dropped, and a new action was started against the Chinese restaurant. The question was: would it be possible to build a concrete case so long after the incident?

It was, of course, impossible to obtain examples of the food that Kim had eaten. And after such a long period of time, she could not remember with great accuracy what she had chosen from the menu. However, I inspected Kim's home kitchen, which was spotlessly clean, and after much legal manoeuvering, was given legal authority to inspect the restaurant conditions. I was not impressed and eventually submitted a report with my colleague, Dr Pat Hayes, in which we stated that there was a 95 per cent certainty that Kim had contracted her illness there.

The Chinese restaurant denied that there was any proof that Kim and her husband had ever been there on the night in question. Despite this, the restaurant's insurers, no doubt fearing a protracted and very expensive court case, plus a great deal of negative publicity, decided to accept liability. On 17 December 1997, almost 11 years after eating that fatal meal, Kim Webb was awarded £1 million in agreed damages for an out-of-court settlement at Manchester High Court.

This was the biggest ever damages award given in a food-poisoning case and it also set an important legal precedent: medical evidence can be taken as proof even if there is no physical evidence remaining of the poisoned food involved. This is significant because it meant that the legal profession and the judiciary were willing to accept science which, for many years, the politicians appeared to dismiss or ignore.

It is cases such as these that the FSA, whose job it will be to police the thousands of restaurants in Britain, will work to try to prevent.

However, these victories have a hollow ring for me. For we are now in the grip of the biggest food-poisoning nightmare of them all, and, as I shall explain next, all my efforts to prevent it were to go unheeded. And – though, unusually for a scientist, I would like to hope that I am wrong – I fear it is too late, now, to stop it.

Part Two

A NATIONAL CATASTROPHE

9

ON THE TRAIL OF THE PRION

In the early 1920s, two German scientists, Doctors Creutzfeldt and Jakob began to research a rare but very unpleasant disease in human beings which, more than half a century later, was to make their names famous throughout the world.

The victims of this disease, mainly people aged between 50 and 70, suffered particularly distressing symptoms. First they would begin to lose muscular coordination which made the most basic functions – walking, the use of their hands, standing up and sitting down – at first difficult and then impossible. Over the passage of a few months, the patients would then begin to shake uncontrollably, their arms, legs and necks twitching non-stop. This shaking was then accompanied by bouts of depression and mania, which included violent temper tantrums and the beating of the head, arms and feet against walls and other solid objects. Eventually, these victims would slip into coma and die. With no known cure, death within a period of some six months from the initial loss of muscular control was inevitable.

Fortunately, the condition was highly unusual, affecting perhaps one in a million people, and at a time when many of the epidemic diseases, such as smallpox, typhoid, TB and diphtheria, were still to be brought largely under control by vaccines and antibiotics, few other medical research centres felt it necessary to devote precious resources to further investigation. When World War Two intervened, the illness, now called Sporadic Creutzfeldt-Jakob disease, or CJD, was virtually ignored except by a handful of scientists who were intrigued by the disease's apparently inexplicable growth.

In their researches, these curious scientists dissected brain tissue from dead victims and found it to be full of tiny holes, rather like a sponge. In other words, it was 'spongiform', or partly rotted away. Just how this had happened, and what had caused it to happen, remained a mystery. The only other similar disease known at the time occurred in sheep:

scrapie, which, like CJD, also has the effect of brain malfunction concerning movement and behaviour, is also slowly progressive, always fatal and untreatable, and also causes changes in the brain with a sponge-like appearance.

Scrapie is a colloquial English name, given because the first symptom shown by affected sheep is that they begin to scrape their legs and hind quarters for hours on end against any hard surface, like a wall or the trunk of a tree. This behaviour becomes so extreme that, eventually, the demented animal rubs away its fleece and then the surface flesh, leaving gaping sores. To observe the progression of such erratic behaviour is distressing for the farmer, because such animals cannot be sent to market and have to be destroyed which, of course, means the loss of hard-earned income. Just how many infected sheep went to market before the disease became apparent is impossible to estimate but, over the century or so when scrapie has been endemic in Britain, it must run in into many thousands, if not tens of thousands.

The attitude to scrapie amongst the British farming community and its mentors in MAFF, is indicative of the 'shrug-of-the-shoulders' approach to veterinary concerns: it was just something that happens from time to time. Very little research was done and affected animals were slaughtered. In other countries, however, curative steps were taken. In Australia and New Zealand, two countries heavily reliant on wool and lamb exports, eradication schemes were launched. Mass slaughter of all affected flocks was initiated, as a result of which, scrapie has now been bred out of these sheep populations. It was this decisive and expensive action that was to take the story into another scientifically intriguing phase.

On the northern tip of the world in the 1940s, the government in Iceland was becoming increasingly concerned about the island's sheep flocks. Iceland is a barren land, dotted with erupting volcanoes and ice floes, and what grazing there is for farm animals is restricted largely to the southern edge of the island. Even this is rarely grass as an English farmer would know it: what vegetation there is largely made up of mosses, lichens, and coarse scrub. Virtually the only possibility of maintaining even a small farming industry was to graze hardy sheep on this subsistence diet. However, scrapie had taken hold on the Icelandic flocks and the entire industry was under threat.

Boldly, the Icelandic authorities decided upon a massive cull: every single sheep from affected flocks was slaughtered and replaced by scrapie-free animals from regions like Australasia. All went well for a few years. Then, much to the dismay of the government and the country's few subsistence shepherds, scrapie began to return. Although this was a major economic setback, the scientific significance of the event was not assimilated then and is still being overlooked today. The inescapable conclusion was that the only way flocks certified to be scrapie-free could have become infected was from the environment. Some infectious agent, as yet still unidentified – which could survive in the open for several years even in those barren Icelandic pastures, some of the most hostile climatic conditions on Earth – had found its way back into healthy sheep. The most likely cause for this is that they ingested it with their food. But no one had the slightest idea what it could be.

The next stage of this saga took place at the other end of the Earth, this time in the dense tropical rain forest of New Guinea. In the 1950s, explorers and anthropologists, closely followed by Christian missionaries, were making first contact with tribes who still used Stone Age technology. These primitive people had no knowledge of the outside world and lived a way of life unchanged for perhaps 20,000 years: hunting, gathering, and fighting occasional wars with the tribes from the next valley in the soaring mountains that cover most of the island.

These people sometimes headhunted, a practice that the missionaries began to stamp out with the help of imported Australian policemen, and also had one habit which was even more disturbing to the white invaders: living in a supremely hostile environment where protein could only be obtained with the greatest of skill and cunning, they wasted nothing. That included human flesh: some of them were cannibals

One tribe in particular attracted the attentions of an American missionary: the Fore (pronounced Foor-ray). All these tribes had differing codes of behaviour but in this one, the men and young boys looked upon cannibalism with disdain. They went out into the jungle on long hunting expeditions and were able to ensure that they were reasonably well fed. The women, largely left behind in their villages of thatched palm huts, were not: and therefore when anyone died, they ate parts of the cadaver and also handled their brains in a strange death ceremony.

The missionary, no doubt appalled and disgusted by this behaviour, began a campaign to stamp out cannibalism. He had noticed one strange occurrence which he used as a weapon in this ideological battle: a much dreaded disease called Kuru which, in the local dialect, means shaking. The curious thing was that Kuru seemed to strike down mainly the women and young children, causing them to lose control of bodily movement, shake violently, and then go into a series of symptoms which ended in mental stupor broken by inexplicable acts of violence. This was followed by pneumonia and death. Only five per cent of cases affected adult men.

This illness set the missionary thinking and he made contact with an American medical research scientist, Dr Carleton Gajdusek, who was so intrigued that he made the long flight to New Guinea. Working in co-operation with a colleague, Dr Zigas, Gajdusek took brain samples from dead Kuru victims and found that certain brain cells, known as neurons, in the area of the brain which controls balance and muscular coordination had been eaten away. By what, he could not say, and it was to be a long time before he could prove that the brain damage was caused by some type of infection. How that infection had arrived in the body, or what type of agent it actually was, was also unknown. For he could find no trace of antibody reaction in the victims.

Here, Gajdusek had stumbled on one of the key difficulties in this entire story. Under normal circumstances when the human body is invaded by infectious agents, either bacteria or viruses, its immune defences quickly identify the type of infection present and begin to produce large quantities of antibodies to kill the invaders. Back in the 1950s, although microbiology was by no means as advanced as it is today, it was fairly straightforward medical practice to identify the different antibodies produced for each infection. Identify the antibody and the infection can also be ascertained. That was the theory then and, in most cases of infection, still is today. Since Gajdusek and Zigas, however, were not able to identify any antibody material, they could not pinpoint the source of the infection.

Writing up their findings (or rather lack of them) in the *New England Journal of Medicine*, in 1957, they recorded that the way in which Kuru affected mainly women and young children – often succeeding generations of the same family – 'supports the suspicion that strong genetic factors are operating'; that is, that something was attacking the genetic make-up of the Fore tribe in a way that affected women and might be passed on to their children. They finished that article with a sentence which, today, rings out like a prophecy: 'If the degeneration of Kuru is a post-infectious phenomenon the antecedent illness must be so mild or subtle as to escape detection by the natives and ourselves.' In layman's language, that means the final, fatal results of Kuru come only a long time after the initial infection. In all illness, early treatment is the best treatment. When Kuru first strikes, it does it so quietly that there are virtually no symptoms to be detected. This, in its turn, makes impossible any early treatment of the disease.

Gajdusek was patently not satisfied with the results of this research and any doctor will know why. He had described the disease, its symptoms and effects, but had not been able to establish beyond doubt that it was, in fact, caused by an infection. The only certain way to show infectivity was by the challenge test. Using brain tissue from Kuru victims, he injected damaged cells into various laboratory animals and found that the disease was transferable to gibbons and several species of monkey from around the world. For this discovery, Gajdusek was eventually awarded the Nobel Prize for Medicine. He had gone a long way to explaining a previously unknown disease but, frustratingly, he had not been able establish the cause of that disease.

That was to not to come until 20 years later.

Although the mysteries surrounding the spread of spongiform brain disease, now widely known as Transmissible Spongiform Encephalopathy or TSE, were of great interest to scientists, they were of little importance to governments or to the world public as a whole. Sporadic CJD was a tragedy when it struck, but, as it infected only one person per million, it could not be looked upon as a major health hazard. Likewise, what government or major drug company was going to pour millions into research to find a cure for Kuru, an illness that affected only one tiny tribe living in one of the world's most remote corners?

Then, in the mid-1960s, something happened that impacted upon big business, and research began in earnest. At that time, before fashions changed and the animal-rights movements began to make themselves felt in the Western world, a mink coat was the ultimate status symbol for the wealthy American woman. The mink had been long hunted almost to extinction in its natural habitats of North America, so the demand for this burgeoning trade in the sixties had been satisfied by mink farming, or ranching, on an industrial scale. By reducing the cost of pelts but by continuing to charge exorbitant prices for the finished product, the mink industry was having a profits bonanza.

Then, throughout the country, mink began to fall ill. Mink are bad-tempered and aggressive creatures at the best of times, but when struck down by this mystery illness, they also went into a form of uncharacteristically and extremely violent dementia which made them almost impossible to handle, and subsequently died. Millions of dollars were at risk, and veterinarians were mobilized in force.

Their first findings showed that the dead animals had a form of TSE: they had spongiform brain cells very similar to those found in scrapie-infected sheep. For some reason, possibly because it sounded far less offensive to the fashion trade than mink scrapie, this disease was given the official name of Transmissible Mink Encephalopathy or TME. Further research showed that many of the dead mink had been fed on cattle offal and other remains from abattoirs. But once again, routine tests could not find the cause of the illness and there was no antibody reaction to give the scientists a clue.

While American mink ranchers howled for a cure, serious-minded scientists concerned with public health had been given some serious food for thought. Here was some sinister new infection on the march, and not only did they not know how it was transmitted, they did not even know what it was. The fact that it had crossed from one species to another set alarm bells ringing in some of North America's leading research establishments: if it could jump from one species to another, were Sporadic CJD and Kuru caused because it could somehow jump into man?

At this time, only six species were known to be susceptible to TSEs under natural conditions: man, with Sporadic CJD and the isolated outbreak of Kuru in New Guinea; sheep; goats; deer; and elk – and now mink. That list was extended artificially during the mink research, when the disease was experimentally transmitted to laboratory animals like mice, rats, hamsters and guinea pigs. It was not known which other species were at risk also: where would that list end?

Even worse, this strange new threat overturned one of the sacred shibboleths of biochemistry. Ever since the secrets of DNA, the so-called building blocks of life, had been unveiled at Cambridge University in 1953 by Nobel Prize winners Francis Crick and J.D. Watson, biochemists had been given a massively powerful tool in their researches. A single strand of DNA, which exists in every living cell, contains all the material to allow that cell to multiply by reproducing an exact replica of itself – a clone, to use the correct term. In helping this reproductive process, DNA also produces a substance called RNA, the material from which the new cells build themselves to the DNA blueprint.

This outstanding (and also British) medical breakthrough had revolutionized medical research into infectious diseases. It had been shown that when a virus invades a body, whether human or animal, the infectious agent uses the host's own DNA and RNA to achieve its own replication. It is in this way that infections like AIDS, herpes and influenza can grow inside the host, sometimes slowly, sometimes at enormous speed. Whilst this very complex process is underway, many proteins are produced as a by-product, proteins that are carried round the body by the blood supply and can, in themselves, be extremely dangerous to the host. Dangerous as they are, however, these proteins are a boon to the doctors searching for the cause of the infection because they can be quickly identified and, like the antibodies, reveal the cause of the illness.

But now, in those minks which had died, there was no trace of these proteins. And that, theoretically at least, meant that the infection did not exist.

Over the next two decades, a scientific brawl ensued. In the United States, the protagonists fell into three camps: one, based at Yale University, insisted that the disease was caused by an as-yet-unknown virus, which was highly resistant to all known treatment; another came up with a micro-organism known as a 'virino', which, it was said, contained an almost immeasurably small particle of DNA or RNA without producing the tell-tale protein by-products; the third was a brilliant scientist, Stanley Prusiner, who put into the language a sinister word that could well have come from the pages of a science-fiction novel: the prion.

During the mink TSE case, researchers had carried out numerous challenge tests on laboratory animals, injecting them with solutions of damaged cells taken from dead mink. Before injection, these cells had been subjected to virtually every weapon known to medicine in attempts to find something that would kill the infection – or whatever was causing the TSE. The solutions, in various strengths, had been heated to temperatures as high as +360°C (well above the required temperature of +70°C for two minutes needed to kill most bacteria). The damaged brain cells were bombarded with X-rays and gamma rays in far larger doses than are ever used in human irradiation treatment. They were dissolved in strong sulphuric acid and in powerful alkaline solutions. They were even burned with blow torches and their ashes, mixed in solution, were injected into the lab animals. Yet each time, the experimental animals were found to be infected by TSE. It was the micro-organism that caused the TSE that Dr Stanley Prusiner named the prion: another 'killer bug', as the newspapers would later say. This one is indestructible by any known medical technique.

Back in the 1950s, Hollywood made a science-fiction film which, despite a B-movie cast, a stilted script and what seemed to be an absurd plot, was destined to become a cult movie. It was called *Invasion of the Body Snatchers*. It told the story of giant seedpods which descended to earth from space and began to take over the world.

The aliens did this by taking over the bodies of human beings, using them as host bodies that would give them the support systems necessary for life on Earth. The hero of the film is a doctor who knows the horrific truth but who, on escaping his invaded hometown, is taken to a psychiatric hospital when he tries to persuade outsiders that such a strange, laughable story could possibly be true.

Prusiner believed that the prion, a tiny particle of protein (unrecognizable to the immune system), could somehow invade an animal's central nervous system. When the prions bury themselves within the host's brain cells, they are not recognized by the body's immune system as an enemy so, unmolested, they begin to breed. Unable to pick up the unwanted presence, the body does not unleash its antibody troops. When a vet or a doctor takes a blood sample, there are no antibodies in the blood, and, therefore, it would appear, there is no disease.

Undetected, prions continue to grow very slowly over a very long period of time – often many years. When they attack the brain, they kill off the individual neurons, the crucial particles responsible for brain function. It is this that creates symptoms such as the inability to control limbs for such simple actions as standing up, or manic rage.

The prion was, Prusiner believed, like the alien from the film – an analogy that is not as far-fetched as it might sound, as events were to prove. But his theory was not to be proved for 20 years.

Whilst the frenzy of research and related controversy was underway in the United States, one more chapter was being added to the TSE story here in Britain. Once again it demonstrated apathy on behalf of the Department of Health and MAFF when it came to protecting the public against potential health hazards from new drugs and medical techniques that, disastrously, had proved not to be properly researched.

Every year, a small number of children are diagnosed as having a medical condition, known by the ugly name of dwarfism, caused by the inability of their pituitary glands to produce natural growth hormones. This only becomes apparent when the children are roughly five years old and their concerned parents begin to realise that they are not growing at a normal rate. This is obviously a distressing condition. So when a drug company came up with a promising solution to the problem, many doctors, parents and indeed the affected children seized upon it with enthusiasm. The newspapers gave this new drug the reassuring name of growth hormone.

What few people outside the medical profession understood was the way in which this growth hormone was gathered. The drug was obtained from the pituitary glands – which are situated directly under the brain and produce hormones responsible for growth – from people who had died either in accidents or from undiagnosed disease. When they were taken into the mortuary, attendants would (usually without relatives' consent) cut out these glands and store them in a refrigerator. When a sufficient supply had been accumulated, they were dispatched to the drug company which processed them to extract the necessary hormones.

The hormones were injected into some 2,000 children at regular intervals over a course of treatment which could last for several years. And the children began to grow, if not to normal height but at least tall enough not to be considered as dwarfs, much to everyone's delight.

The euphoria was not to last long. By the end of the 1980s, when the existence of the prion was first being suggested by medical science, children who had undergone growth-hormone treatment were beginning to suffer from strange, serious illnesses. They began to stagger and lose their memory, then become demented before slipping into a coma. Then came the first of some 30 deaths amongst growth-hormone patients. Brain samples showed that the youngsters were suffering from a disease similar to CJD. Another variant had been added to this sad human condition which, only a few decades earlier, had been restricted to the unfortunate one-in-a-million human being. It is not yet known what effects the treatment might have on the offspring of those who underwent it.

The growth-hormone disaster was to raise many more important questions than it answered. Just why a human pituitary gland (and possibly transplanted organs) can be the source of a CJD infection is not yet clear. Could it mean that prions are present there naturally in minute quantities, as yet undetected, in most people? Had the postmortem subjects been harbouring CJD but died before the disease had time to take hold (indeed, it is not clear why all potential recipients of abnormal prions do not succumb to CJD infection)? If so, where had that infection come from?

What was not known at the time was that the prion was marching through the shires of England in the form of BSE, slowly but surely invading the brains of thousands of cattle, who began to suffer from Mad Cow Disease.

We did not know then that this new strain of spongiform disease, BSE, could be passed to humans. But without doubt, as I shall show, a human form of BSE was already in our food chain. That, I suggest, is how youngsters who undertook growth-hormone treatment were infected: by prions which were already at work in the bodies of people who had ingested them with the Beef of Olde England.

10

DUPED

In the mid-years of the 1980s, I was so involved in other food-poisoning scandals that I took little notice of the reports that began to emerge in 1986 of cows going mad in the countryside. I was aware, of course, that the emergence of a scrapie-like disease in cattle meant that, somehow, this disease or a similar one had crossed another species barrier but, as my main role was in the field of human health, I did not immediately perceive a threat to people.

However, from 1986 onwards, I did have a secondary role which impinged on veterinary matters as a member of the MAFF Veterinary Products Committee. My place on this came about because, just before the Stanley Royd Hospital disaster, I and various colleagues at Leeds had carried out a lengthy piece of research into the growing resistance to some well-known antibiotics amongst infectious bacteria.

The problem of immunity in bacteria was by no means so acute in Britain as elsewhere but, by the mid-1980s, there were signs that it was growing here, too. No one was quite sure why. Suspicion was beginning to fall on the widespread use of veterinary antibiotics fed to livestock, poultry and even to farmed salmon. As often as not, large doses were being administered not to cure a disease which had already taken hold but as a preventive to avoid possible outbreaks in the future. Amongst doctors, concern was increasing that these often unnecessary doses were entering the human food chain and, as a result, were bringing about increased antibiotic resistance in bacteria which cause illness in people.

This was at the time when I was based in Kings Lynn, Norfolk, working for the East Anglia Health Authority, and my department was asked to research this issue with funds provided by the American pharmaceutical company, Eli Lilly. We launched a five-year investigation and our findings, published in scientific journals and books, cleared veterinary antibiotics as the main cause of increased bacterial resistance in humans. On the contrary, we discovered that the cause was more likely to have been the over-prescription of human antibiotics by doctors to patients who could have been treated with other drugs less likely to create long-term problems.

One of the effects of these findings was that, for the first and only time in my life, I became something of a darling to the vets and their farmer customers (a situation which might cause some wry smiles today). As a result, I was asked to join the MAFF Veterinary Products Committee. The committee was made up of some of the best-known names in medicine and veterinary science, and its role was to advise the government on possible public health hazards resulting from many of the rapid changes underway in British farm production. These included, not just antibiotics, but hormones given to livestock to increase growth rates, new feedstuffs being developed, and any potential threat to human health from intensive-rearing practices such as battery poultry- and pig-farming.

I have to admit that I felt honoured to be asked to join this group. Here, I believed, my advice would be listened to by senior civil servants who, in turn, reported directly to the Minister of Agriculture. I was to be given the ear of the government at a time when the first murmurings of unrest were being raised about the safety of new methods of food production, processing and cooking. Here, I thought, was an opportunity to influence food policy directly in the best interests of the British public.

I now believe, because of the subsequent events I shall describe, that I had been offered the job because the results of our veterinary antibiotic research had been what the government, or at least its MAFF underlings, had wanted. Had the research gone the other way, I would have been anathema to the people I now joined as a valued colleague.

For a couple of years, I believed, or perhaps deceived myself, that this committee was doing a good job in the interests of both the farmers and the food-consuming public. Then the doubts began to set in.

The committee was composed of some 20 or so eminent specialists – vets, doctors, scientists – but I soon became increasingly irritated by the behaviour of a group of MAFF civil servants who always sat in a group at the bottom of the long committee table. Officially, these civil servants were not members of the committee. Their role, allegedly, was to offer advice when requested and to take notes of any decisions made in order to report our recommendations back to the Minister of Agriculture, Mr

John MacGregor. But instead of taking a passive role, the group regularly interrupted meetings with vacuous, and often misleading, information. If anything positive was ever achieved, it was usually done in face of their hindrance rather than with the help they were supposedly there to provide. It took me some time to realize that many Whitehall mandarins believe in the maxim that the best action to take in most given situations is no action at all.

The chairman of the committee was a distinguished vet, Professor James Armour, who was later to be knighted. Armour was Dean of the Veterinary School at Glasgow University, that prestigious school which included the writer James Herriot and many other famous vets amongst its graduates. With Margaret Thatcher slashing away at public spending like a pirate with a cutlass, it was under threat of closure. This put Armour in a highly invidious position: he was supposed to be advising the government whilst wearing one hat and fighting it whilst donning the other. He also had my presence on his committee to contend with.

Although I had been invited to join as a result of my research, the vets' gratitude quickly evaporated because of the public stances I took in the salmonella and listeria scandals. Also, most vets, with some honourable exceptions, tend to work very closely with their farmer customers, and to my eyes, most judge the interests of vets and farmers to be the same. On a committee whose purpose was to protect the public against any possible threat from new farm practices or drugs, I found this unacceptable. (Although to condemn a whole profession must be a generality, I still do: in the traumas that were to follow, most vets automatically sided with MAFF interests long after it was becoming clear that human health was at risk.) Inevitably, as my sense of disillusionment grew, there were spats.

I have no doubt that there were many people at MAFF, and even other members of the committee, who would have dearly loved to see me sacked from the Veterinary Products Committee, because I became a thorn in their side. However, I was by now a well-known media figure after the salmonella debacle and the listeria campaign. To have dismissed me would have invited yet more headlines and yet another scandal. To use the late President Johnson's crude but striking analogy, they would rather have me in the tent pissing out than outside pissing in.

One of the spats, I believe, illustrates the reluctance of the committee to recommend any course of action which, although in the public interest, might conflict with commercial needs. In the mid-1980s, salmon farming had become a growth industry in northern Britain, providing many thousands of jobs in small coastal towns where traditional fishing was in steep decline. This marvellous fish, which has one of the most remarkable lifecycles in the animal kingdom, was trapped and then bred in millions in stationary cages suspended in sea lochs. As with intensive chicken farming, this had the effect of drastically reducing the price of this once-luxury delicacy: salmon very quickly became cheaper than haddock or cod, which pleased the producers, the supermarket owners and, no doubt, their customers.

However, as far as I am aware, no one had studied in detail the effects of this stationary existence on a previously wild animal. Salmon, of course, start their lives as an egg in the rushing rivers and burns of Scotland, go to sea as a young parr no longer than your hand, and return to breed in their home river one, two or even four years later as a mature fish weighing up to 18kg (40lb): not for nothing do anglers call the salmon the king of fish. Those same anglers would also have told MAFF officials, had they ever been asked, that even wild salmon can suffer from infestations of lice, which grow on their bodies and suck their blood. These sea lice die in fresh water and drop off a few days after the salmon has entered its home river – so anglers know that the presence of a few lice on a mature salmon's silver body mean that the fish is 'fresh run'. To the fisherman, the presence of sea lice means that the fish is absolutely fresh from the sea and therefore the finest catch a British game angler can ever make.

Farmed fish were kept all their lives in salt water, the natural environment of the lice. Presented with these tens of thousands of farmed salmon hopelessly trapped in their cages, the lice went into an explosion of replication. In nature, fish can act as host to a handful of lice without undue damage to their health, but they were now being covered by hundreds of them. Not only did the lice suck the salmon's blood in ever-growing quantities, which obviously weakened the fish, but they also left ugly scars on its silvery skin. This did not please the supermarkets, for the fish, laid out in their glory on the fishmonger's slab, seemed disfigured – and no one would buy them.

The fish farmers, threatened with bankruptcy, knew that something had to be done. Then, someone, somewhere – nobody knows quite who it was, officially at least – discovered that an organophosphate used in sheep dips to kill ticks and other pests was also effective against sea lice. Without authority, without specialist scientific advice and without any data proving its safety – thus in breach of the Medicines Act 1968, which requires a product to be of suitable quality, efficacy and safety to those who use or are exposed to it – the producers began to dose their fish with sheep dip in open water, an act of environmental stupidity so gross that it almost defies belief. Just to throw away an empty dip tin can attract large fines, for if any residue leaches into the water table, it can cause immense damage to fish and insect life in streams and rivers. On farms, sheep dipping must be done in properly maintained, concrete-lined pits, which are inspected regularly to ensure they are leak-proof. Moreover, shepherds must wear proper breathing equipment when dipping sheep, or risk serious poisoning: there are now several cases before the courts of farmers allegedly brain-damaged by these potent chemicals.

Yet here on the west coast of Scotland, in what had once been some of the clearest and most pollution-free stretches of salt water on the entire coast of the British Isles, salmon farmers were indiscriminately dumping unrecorded amounts of these deadly chemicals into the open sea.

Slowly but inevitably, reports of this activity filtered down to MAFF in London and, eventually, to the Veterinary Products Committee. The day before we were due to meet to discuss this issue, a delegation of Scottish salmon farmers – most of whom, in fact, were English – paid a call on MAFF. They must be given legal permission to continue using organophosphates, they said, or they would go out of business. Thousands of people would be thrown out of work in the remoter areas of Scotland. Whether or not they said failure to give this permission would cost the Conservatives Scottish seats at the next general election I cannot say, but I have no doubt whatsoever that this was a problem large in the minds of the political masters at MAFF.

I did not know about this when I sat down for the meeting. As far as I was concerned, this was an open-and-shut case: the salmon producers had been acting illegally and with total contempt of the most basic environmental considerations. Under the Veterinary Product Committee's own rules, only products which had been proved to be effective and without side effects in one species could be used on another similar species. To suggest that a salmon is similar to a sheep would take us into Alice's Wonderland. The salmon producers, I thought, would not only be refused permission to continue using organophosphates but, if justice were to be done, should also be recommended for prosecution.

It was all over in minutes. A motion was put that the approved use of sheep dips should be extended to salmon. Before I even had chance to speak, the chairman called for a vote. Every hand went up but mine. 'Anyone against?' asked the chairman. I was the solitary objector.

This was one of the key committees that would, a few years later, advise government on the biggest food-poisoning crisis in history.

After the salmon fiasco, my faith in the Veterinary Products Committee to do anything more than rubber-stamp government action already decided – as opposed to providing essential scientific advice on which future policy could be reliably based – disintegrated. I did stay on, however, for another year or so. I still clung to a vague hope that I might be able to accomplish something useful in the public interest; and it enabled me to be privy to technical information which was not made widely available to the general public and, as a scientist, information is my life blood.

This was important, for soon I became more and more absorbed by the implications of a disease that, at that point, was outside my professional remit. In November 1986, the first cases of TSE were confirmed in British cattle. At least, these were the first admitted cases. It was to emerge 12 years later that a case of 'cattle scrapie' had been confirmed a year before, but had been filed away and forgotten. Thanks to MAFF intervention, this new disease was not to be called cattle scrapie – that might be distasteful in the consumer's eye; as in the American mink outbreak, it was given the biologically correct name of Bovine Spongiform Encephalopathy or BSE, a name that was soon to become as familiar to the man in the street as the more emotive Mad Cow Disease.

Although largely overlooked, at the same time a similar disease was reported in an antelope at Marwell Zoo, Hampshire. Two more species had been added to the growing list of animals known to be naturally susceptible, as opposed to laboratory animals into which diseased tissue had been injected under experimental conditions.

I was, like millions of other Britons, duped. This is something no one likes to admit but I believed the MAFF and Department of Health statements that poured scorn on the idea that this disease could spread to humans, arguing that as sheep scrapie had been known for generations without any major threat to human health, so BSE would be the same. At first, without any evidence to the contrary, I was satisfied that this was a veterinary problem, not a medical one.

In October 1987, the first scientific paper on BSE was published in the *Veterinary Record*. This confirmed that it was a spongiform disease, which we already knew, and that its cause was unknown, which we also knew. But by now I was becoming increasingly concerned that few routine precautions were being taken to protect human health, just in case the disease was transferable to humans. I did not know that certain vets were already telling MAFF officials that there might be a danger to human health. Those vets were persuaded to keep this view to themselves, unfortunately: just one veterinary whistle-blower at this point might have nipped in the bud a growing health threat of almost incalculable proportions. The Public Health Laboratory Service was deliberately excluded.

It was evident in 1987 that infected carcasses were entering the human food chain via the abattoirs. They were also going into food for domestic pets, zoo animals, and farm livestock and poultry being bred specifically for human consumption. This realization began to awaken my first real fears, because I knew only too well the ease with which infections, even unknown ones, enter the human body in the food we eat. By the end of 1987, 420 cases of BSE had been reported throughout the United Kingdom, and the epidemic was obviously spreading very quickly. But no government action had been taken to make it a 'notifiable disease' – a disease which, by law, a farmer must report to the local MAFF vet.

This alarmed me. There is a very long list of notifiable farm diseases including foot-and mouth-disease, swine fever, TB in cows, and blue-eared pig disease. When these are reported, travel restrictions are imposed almost immediately. Infected animals cannot be sold from one farm to another, or taken to market, for fear of spreading the disease. In foot-and-mouth, which wipes out huge numbers of cattle but is not usually dangerous to humans, infected animals are usually destroyed on their home farm and incinerated in pits there and then, so seriously is it taken. TB-infected milk, which had killed thousands of people in Britain over many generations, had been virtually eradicated after World War Two by the simple process of pasteurization. Yet here was a new disease with severe effects, its cause unknown, and the government was doing virtually nothing to stop its spread.

By 1988, the government, hitherto unwilling to take any form of action with regard to BSE, set up a committee. Its role was to consider, amongst other issues, whether there was 'any possible' hazard to public health from BSE.

As always, this committee boasted an impressive list of members whose names were, presumably, meant to reassure the public of their scientific excellence and independence. The chairman was Professor Sir Richard Southwood, then Linacre Professor of Zoology at Oxford University. Other members included Professor M.A. Epstein, Emeritus Professor of Pathology, Bristol University; Dr W.B. Martin, formerly Director of the Moredun research Institute in Edinburgh, and Sir John Walton, formerly Professor of Neurology at Newcastle University. (Following the publication of their report a year later, Sir Richard was promoted to Vice Chancellor at Oxford, Professor Epstein was knighted and Sir John became Lord Walton.)

I was delighted that something was being done and that there would be an in-depth investigation of BSE and its possible dangers to humans. What troubled me, however, was that none of these men, as far as I could ascertain, had ever done any research work into spongiform diseases. No experts in this field were ever co-opted onto the committee; nor did the committee call evidence from American scientists like Prusiner and Gajdusek, the acknowledged world experts in the field. In other words, the composition of the committee seemed to me like sending a cricket umpire to referee a rugby match.

While the committee sat, more and more scientists began to put forward what to me is the key question about all potential risks to public health. Government policy seemed thus far to have been driven by the attitude that minimal action was required until it was proved that BSE could be passed to humans in one form or another. My point, which many other people now echoed, was the opposite: that until it could be proved beyond doubt that this could *not* happen, and that there was no danger, all possible precautions should be taken to exclude diseased carcasses from the human food chain.

In June, 1988, the *British Medical Journal* published a paper by Dr Tim Holt, a junior doctor in a London hospital, and a colleague J. Phillips. This pointed out that, as BSE was a spongiform disease, and as humans were known to be susceptible to spongiform diseases such as CJD and Kuru, there was a possibility that humans might also be vulnerable to BSE. This was the first time such a possibility had been aired in a responsible medical journal and it caused many critical comments in the media.

Also that month, the then Health Secretary, Kenneth Clarke, admitted that infected meat had found its way into the human food chain. Public reaction to this confession was, understandably, extremely hostile and the government was forced into further action. On 20 June, the Southwood Committee made its first serious recommendation: that until more was known about BSE, the carcasses of affected animals should be destroyed. The government appeared to assimilate the fact that they had a growing problem on their hands. In a step in the right direction, the following month – two years after BSE had first been officially isolated in cattle but three since the first reported case – the Minister of Agriculture, John MacGregor, accepted the Southwood recommendations and issued a press release that read: 'Pending the final conclusion of the working party, arrangements will be made for compulsory slaughter and destruction of carcasses. Compensation will be payable at 50 per cent of market value subject to a ceiling.'

For the first time, the government began to open the public purse in a belated attempt to remedy a situation that it would have avoided had it acted earlier. Estimates of the final bill to the British taxpayer are impossible to calculate, for if there is the large-scale outbreak of human CJD in the first half of the twenty-first century, which I fear is almost inevitable, the medical costs will be astronomical. By early 1998, the cost to the taxpayer is already estimated to have passed the £2 billion mark and is still rising. The cost to the British beef industry is probably much the same in lost sales. Moreover, it was this first offer of 50 per cent compensation which, in many opinions other than my own, sowed the seeds of this financial disaster.

The reason is that such a decision put grave temptation before the farming community. The vast majority of these men and women are, of course, honest, hard-working folk with large sums of capital invested in their farms. All were becoming increasingly concerned at the gathering crisis and the threat it presented to their future livelihoods. So how many were tempted, when spotting the first symptoms in their herds, to dump those animals on the market before the symptoms became so obvious as to make the animal unsaleable? This is another unanswerable question, but it would be reasonable to assume that after the slaughter policy was announced many hundreds of cows went to market whose owners knew that they had already been carrying the disease for many months, perhaps even years. Had the government decided to pay out 100 per cent compensation, it would not have solved the problem entirely but might have prevented the fact that many human beings are now carrying in their bodies prions from cattle which would otherwise have been slaughtered and buried or burned. More important than the cost issue is the fact that this decision came too late to have prevented BSE – either to the farmers' knowledge or not – from entering the human food chain.

Having recommended the slaughter policy, the Southwood committee also made another suggestion that was, in effect, an admission of its own inability to understand the scientific implications of the problem. It sought the creation of yet another committee, which it could consult on the intricacies of the research being undertaken into BSE and similar spongiform diseases. Had the right people been selected in the first place, this would have been unnecessary. So in June 1988, the Southwood Committee begat the Tyrrell Committee – more properly called the Spongiform Encephalopathy Advisory Committee, or SEAC – under the chairmanship of Dr David Tyrrell, a former Director of the Medical Council's Common Cold Unit! Dr Tyrrell, CBE, is without doubt an eminent doctor but what, many people might ask, is the connection between the common cold and a killer disease spread by unknown means by unknown organisms? The only similarity I can think of is that both, at present, are incurable.

The Southwood Committee then retired for a long summer break and did not meet again until November. In the meantime, the government took another important step by banning the feeding of animal proteins to ruminants, meaning grazing animals such as cattle, sheep, goats and deer.

Apart from its importance in eliminating a possible method of spreading BSE, this decision has hidden ramifications, for it was the first tacit admission that there might be something amiss in forcing herbivorous animals to become carnivores. There are many people who have deep-felt moral or even religious objections to this process. For the religious, it flies in the face of God-given laws. For the growing number of people turning to vegetarianism and veganism, it is a moral outrage. I too feel this moral indignation about defenceless animals being forced into unnatural practices but, as a scientist, I have more deeply seated professional concerns.

At the beginning of this book, I put forward the hypothesis that many of the food-poisoning outbreaks of recent years came about as a result of mankind discarding cooking practices that killed harmful bacteria. Over hundreds of generations, the human body has become accustomed to the ingestion of cooked food – most people forced to eat raw meat would now vomit or suffer serious stomach disorders. Over the millennia, the human body had reached a balance whereby its bodily defences could cope with most of the infections it was likely to face. When we began to discard traditional cooking and food-storage methods, we exposed ourselves to new threats with which our natural defences were unable to cope.

Likewise, over millions of years of evolution ruminants had developed finely balanced bodily mechanisms which permitted them to thrive, in Britain at least, on a diet that consisted mainly of grasses, shoots and, occasionally, leaves. Internally, their antibody mechanisms had become fine-tuned to deal with any pests or bacteria that they were likely to ingest whilst grazing. Obviously, animals, like humans, become ill from time to time but, by and large, the ruminants were and are highly successful species.

Then twentieth-century man decided that he could ignore that balance and overturn natural processes. And the reason for this act of brazen arrogance: commercial greed.

It was discovered that, when even the the most unsavoury cuts of meat had been used for human consumption in items like pies and sausages, the slaughterhouses still had large quantities of animal tissue in need of disposal: the coarsest offals, skin, gristle, ears, noses, and many bones. Disposal was difficult and expensive. Some went into bone meal for gardeners, but much of it had to be incinerated, which is both costly and, increasingly, environmentally unacceptable. Then someone had the bright idea that much of it could be cooked – 'rendered' in the trade term – and ground up into animal feed. Here was every agri-businessman's dream: as in the case of feeding poultry to poultry, described earlier, a waste material could be reused, saving on disposal costs; and it could also be turned into another profitable line of production.

They argued, at the beginning, that many farm animals do have quantities of meat protein in their natural diets. Pigs will eat almost anything, animal or vegetable, and even goats have been known to eat carrion. Poultry, too, have quite large amounts of animal protein in their diets, from carrion, waste from human kitchens, and – if they are lucky to live in a farmyard where they can scratch about for food – any worms or insects they can catch. Under normal circumstances, if the animal protein they are fed is not actually diseased, these animals and their bodily defence mechanisms can cope. Then someone discovered, probably to his surprise, that ruminants could be fed animal protein too.

This practice of feeding animal proteins to cattle began in the mid-twentieth-century. It soon became standard practice with no apparent side effects. Although it was not public knowledge – had it been, it would no doubt have caused a wave of revulsion – under this practice the remains of slaughtered sheep known to be victims of scrapie were routinely treated and sold on as animal feed.

On this issue, I find myself in conflict with the attitudes of the veterinary profession, who were aware of this practice. When these processes were underway, I have no doubt that most vets believed that, in the rendering and grinding up of scrapie-riddled sheep, all potentially harmful infectious agents would be killed. This belief, to me, contains a serious flaw on ethical and perhaps moral grounds but also flies in the face of all accepted medical and veterinary practice: when faced with disease, one should automatically do everything possible to prevent its spread. That most certainly does not include feeding diseased remains, however well processed, to other creatures.

What concerned me most, however, was that the ban on feeding animal proteins to ruminants was misguided as a preventive measure against the spread of BSE, because it was based on the belief that BSE was in fact scrapie. I would not expect the vets who advised the government to be familiar with the occurrences of Kuru disease in New Guinea. I would, however, have expected them to be aware of the existence of Sporadic Creutzfeldt-Jakob disease which was, like BSE, a spongiform disease, and therefore, as Dr Tim Holt and J. Phillips had pointed out, possibly linked to BSE. Since Sporadic CJD had never, in more than 70 years of research, shown any particular association with sheep, and since scrapie had been known in Britain for almost two centuries without any quantifiable risks to human health, the belief that BSE was basically scrapie that had crossed the species barrier, and was therefore harmless to humans, was a suspect assumption. I was beginning to smell the distinctive odour of red herring.

An additional point here is that knowledgeable scientists who had studied the history of spongiform diseases in both humans and animals would have been struck by some coincidences. Just as Kuru in New Guinea seemed to be closely linked with cannibalism, so in the American mink outbreak, living animals had also been known to eat dead victims of the disease, another act of cannibalism. And while some of the artificial feed fed to cattle since the 1960s was known to come from sheep, the vast majority was from cattle. So, cattle had become cannibals too. Could there be a link here? If there is – and it has still not been established, because virtually no research is being done in this direction – BSE comes from infected *beef* in animal feed, not mutton, so disproving again the linking of BSE to scrapie.

Whether or not the vets have considered this possibility, I do not know. I do know, however, that by persuading the public that BSE was in fact a form of scrapie, MAFF had reassured them that, as scrapie was no threat to humans, they were, *ipso facto*, safe from BSE, and the removal of diseased sheep and cattle from the human food chain was merely a wise and possibly unnecessary precaution. This link, however, was based on the flimsiest of evidence, and was therefore in effect a smoke screen. For a year or so, it was extremely effective in obscuring the truth.

11

THE BIG LIE

In February 1989, a Big Lie was foisted upon the British public. It was contained in a three-word phrase: 'dead-end host'.

The phrase was first used in public when the Southwood Committee published its investigations into the threat to human health caused by BSE. In many ways, this report was a well-meaning document and for the vast majority of its length, it discussed the scientific confusion over the spread of the disease with openness and honesty.

It admitted that 'conflicting evidence has been accumulated' about the possibility that sheep scrapie could be a source of CJD in humans. There was no evidence to support the suggestion that the disease could be spread orally to humans by eating diseased sheep organs. And it added: 'Scrapie has been endemic in Britain for centuries without there being evidence to show an incidence of CJD higher than the international average in the human population.'

Now this last point was designed, no doubt, to reassure the public that as scrapie had not been proved dangerous to humans, BSE – still thought by many to be a bovine form of scrapie – was also harmless. But there is a flaw here: even if scrapie could not spread to humans, what evidence was there that it could spread to cattle?

It went on to discuss the various spongiform diseases in animals and humans and admitted that mice injected with diseased cells from BSE cattle had developed similar symptoms over a period of ten to eleven months, which is an extremely long period in the lifetime of a mouse. When infected, these laboratory mice inevitably died and, when diseased cells from these dead mice were injected into further experimental animals in challenge tests, this second batch also developed the symptoms. Comparing the fast growth of the disease in injected animals, it also pointed out sombrely that in Kuru cases, such symptoms could take as long as 30 years to develop in human beings.

The report added: 'In summary, the present state of knowledge shows that all these diseases have similar pathologies with spongiform change in the central nervous system ... They are inevitably fatal and the causal subviral agents are not destroyed by normal sterilisation processes.'

This was a confession of just how little we knew about BSE at the time. In referring to 'causal subviral agents' it admits that something is spreading this disease, but what it is we do not know. In saying that this agent, whatever it is, is 'not destroyed by normal sterilisation processes' it admits that even if we knew what this mystery invader was, we still had no defences against it. In other words, here was a fatal disease with no known cause and no known cure. This was the same conclusion that had been reached in North America almost 25 years earlier during the outbreak of spongiform brain disease in mink.

Predicting the future course of the disease, Southwood looked into a crystal ball and suggested that at the then growth rate of BSE cases, some 17,000 to 20,000 cattle were likely to have been infected before the disease was largely eradicated in 1993 and finally wiped out by 1996. (The actual figures, in March, 1998, show that some 160,000 cattle have in fact contracted the disease and, although the rate of infection is said to be declining, it is far from being eradicated.)

Though that comment was proved wrong, there was one passage in the report, perhaps the most chilling of all, which still holds true today. It said: 'With the very long incubation period of spongiform encephalopathies in humans, it may be a decade or more before complete reassurance can be given.'

This was a classic piece of fence-sitting. The Southwood Committee had been appointed to provide a balanced judgement on the possible dangers of BSE to human health. This sentence was an admission that it could not make such a judgement. Unwilling, at this stage of the report at least, to make predictions which might prove drastically wrong, the committee allowed themselves an escape hatch.

Had the government adopted the view, as I and others did, that all possible precautions should be taken against the spread of BSE into the human food chain until it could be proved conclusively that it posed no threat to human health, this single sentence should have been enough to bring about massive government action. There should have been an immediate slaughter policy of all cattle herds in which BSE had occurred, which at the time was running in the order of 350 to 400 a month. There should have been a joint medical and veterinary research programme launched, similar to the one which was then tackling the AIDS problem.

But this was 1989, the year that the Thatcher bubble was about to burst, when the Thatcher economic miracle was to hit the wall, sending unemployment soaring and leaving hundreds of thousands of young couples unable to pay the mortgages on homes worth less than what they had paid for them. With soaring unemployment increasing the cost of social security and decreasing tax revenues, any thought of a multi-million-pound payout by the treasury for the slaughter of cattle herds was out of the question.

Therefore the Southwood report did little to assuage public demand for action in a situation of the greatest anxiety and had little effect until its very last page. That, I believe, is when the Big Lie came into play.

The ultimate conclusion of the Southwood report read:

From present evidence, it is likely that cattle will prove to be a 'dead-end host' for the disease agent and most unlikely that BSE will have any implications for human health. Nevertheless, if our assessment of these likelihoods is incorrect, the implications would be extremely serious.

Thus, we greatly welcome the speed with which the Ministry of Agriculture, Fisheries and Food has brought forward regulations based on the veterinary evidence and on our recommendations, and are encouraged by what we have learned of the positive response from the animal foods and farming industries to ensure the effectiveness of the regulations.

These two paragraphs contain, as I will show, an honest piece of scientific doubt, a statement which is blatantly contradictory to many of the findings in the earlier, more detailed passages of the report, and concludes with a classic passage of civil service gobbledygook which hands MAFF a generous pat on the back in a situation that in my view was completely unwarranted.

Most scientists should go into public print only after carrying out experimental work which satisfies tightly drawn criteria that their findings have been proved correct. That the first paragraph uses the words include 'likely' in relation to the 'dead-end host' theory and 'unlikely' in relation to its threat to human health shows that the scientists on the committee were unable to prove their findings correct. That sense of uncertainty is reinforced by the admission that 'if our assessments of these likelihoods are incorrect, the implications would be extremely serious.' One does not have to be a skilled cryptologist to see that these words are code which really mean: 'We are keeping our fingers crossed and hoping we are right'.

The phrase 'dead-end host' means that the infectious agent attacking BSE-infected cattle will stay within cattle and not jump into another species. This contradicts the earlier passages of the report which confirm that the disease had infected mice under laboratory conditions. So cows are not a dead-end host, for the fact that mice can contract the disease, admittedly under experimental conditions, suggests that it might be possible for other species to be infected. So, by its own admission, the dead-end host theory is open to doubt, and no evidence was given in the report to prove it. The Big Lie came about because the government interpreted and broadcast the theory as truth.

There are other sinister implications revealed earlier in the report. It detailed efforts being made by the Health and Safety Executive to alert farmers, slaughtermen and other workers regularly in contact with cattle against the dangers of possible BSE infection from handling the placenta of newborn calves from BSE-infected mothers. It was known that scrapie was found in the placenta, and it was theoretically possible that infection from cattle placenta could enter the human body through abrasions in the skin. Yet at this time – and for many years later – no government scientist ever admitted the possibility that BSE could be spread by downward transmission: i.e., from mother to calf. Such an admission would have created a demand for an even wider-spread slaughter policy for, officially at least, calves born after the ban on feeding animal proteins to cattle were judged to be free of risk from BSE.

Here we have an example of government doublespeak: cows could not pass the disease down to their offspring – yet their placentas, and therefore inevitably their calves, might be infected. And if the disease cannot be passed to humans through beef, why should this precaution be taken anyway?

Civil servants would, no doubt, argue that this was just another largely unnecessary additional safety measure, just in case. But the very fact that this advice was issued by the Health and Safety Executive shows, on the public record, that someone, somewhere believed that such a risk existed, even if in theory only. Unfortunately, these contradictions in a lengthy report went largely unnoticed by the media. Their attention was directed, by politicians and their skilled spin doctors, to the dead-end host theory, which was to be trotted out again and again in the coming months and years. To members of the scientific community, however, the uncertainties and contradictions in the Southwood Report set off an ever-widening circle of concern. It was as I read the report time and time again, concentrating on the scientific content, that I began to form a suspicion that the vital conclusion of the report, the dead-end host theory, was in conflict with its scientific evidence.

As I write this in the spring of 1998, the enquiry into the BSE debacle set up by Labour Minister of Agriculture, Dr Jack Cunningham, is taking place. For the first time, scientists and vets employed by the previous Conservative administration are coming forward to explain publicly some of the background to decisions taken behind closed doors.

One of the emerging fragments of this complex tale is the fact that, when the Southwood Report was being prepared for publication, there was warfare between the Department of Health and MAFF on the final wording. Such was this feuding that a Department of Health mandarin actually delivered what was to be the final draft to members of the committee on Christmas Eve 1989, so that they could study it over the Christmas period without pressure from MAFF officials. It was some time in the New Year before MAFF knew that the final draft was even in preparation.

The key question here, which the enquiry committee has now asked, is: was the Southwood Report's final conclusion changed at the last minute by some politician or civil servant? All the members (Southwood, Epstein, Martin and Walton) agreed to the statement 'From present evidence, it is likely that cattle will prove to be a dead-end host for the disease agent and most unlikely that BSE will have any implications for human health.' Epstein alone inserted the next sentence,

'Nevertheless, if our assessments of these likelihoods are incorrect, the implications would be extremely serious.'

By implying that the disease was not infectious, the Big Lie set back the course of BSE research for years. During that time, hundreds, perhaps thousands, of people continued to eat beef that was still infected with BSE despite the ban on animal cattle feed, for although it was not proved until later – and the idea was vehemently denied by dozens of politicians and government PR people, despite the Health and Safety Executive admitting that it was a possibility – in fact the disease was being passed down from mother to calf by vertical transmission. It is therefore highly likely that some of these consumers are already infected with BSE, the infection growing slowly but inexorably in their bodies before attacking their central nervous systems.

Sadly, the Southwood Report had the effect that was intended. Parliament, the media and the public accepted the dead-end host theory and consumers went on about their business as usual. In the countryside, the disease continued to spread, causing great distress and financial loss in rural communities, to which in the towns and big cities people were generally unsympathetic. Over many generations, the farmers had developed in urban eyes an image of a pampered, subsidized, over-influential minority who were always complaining however much money they earned. This, in fact, was a distortion of the truth, but one which was to cost the agriculture industry much public support in the years to come – support which it could ill-afford to lose.

One evening at the end of 1989, I was invited to take part in a televised debate on Channel 4 on BSE and its risks to people, alongside Tim Holt, the young hospital doctor who had first voiced medical fears more than 12 months earlier about the potential of BSE spreading to humans. Officially at least, his fears had been contradicted by the Southwood Report. But it was well known in the public health world that Tim had been subjected to considerable criticism from both political and health service sources for choosing to speak out. Some said that his entire future career was in the balance. With considerable courage, he had decided to stick by his guns.

In some flight of creative fancy, this debate took place in a tent, presumably to give the impression that we were in a rural setting, perhaps at an agricultural show. On the other side of the debate were representatives from MAFF and the farming industry who, for the entire length of the discussion, poured scorn on every suggestion made by Tim and myself. Whilst not actually on camera, I watched these people with studied interest. They were so emphatic with their denials, so certain of 'facts' which were scientifically unproven, that it seemed to me that they were working to a prepared script, perfectly rehearsed. Despite this, their body language and off-camera fidgeting suggested to me that they were far less convinced by their case. It seemed to me that, in Shakespeare's words spoken in different circumstances, 'The lady doth protest too much'.

After the programme, one of the MAFF men came up and looked me rather shamed-facedly in the eye. 'Sorry about that, Professor,' he said, 'But that was the line we had been ordered to take.'

That was the moment when all the doubts of the last three years came to a head. Until then, I had believed that BSE was a largely veterinary problem, albeit an extremely difficult one. I went home that night convinced, by instinct, even if I did not yet have the evidence, that something much more serious was afoot: that the government was already in possession of evidence which it was covering up. And because of my continued membership of the Veterinary Products Committee, I felt that I could not speak out and that I was condoning that cover-up. That situation was soon to resolve itself.

In the autumn of 1989, the Veterinary Products Committee was considering a new cattle hormone called BST which, when injected into cows, greatly increased their milk yields. Vets and the drug companies were eager to get permission to use this new drug despite the fact that, at this time, the then-EEC was wrestling with the problems of over-production. Europe was awash with milk lakes and butter mountains, and most serious-minded politicians were putting their minds to ways of reducing milk production. Not so MAFF.

Although I could see no acceptable political or economic grounds for putting BST into wholesale use, my main objections, which I made to the committee, were on medical and veterinary grounds. The government had admitted that whatever the risks to human health, BSE had become a major veterinary plague: their own figures were predicting a death rate of 17,000 to 20,000 but, within months of that estimate being published, almost everyone involved accepted that they were a hopeless underestimate. And no one knew how the disease was being transmitted. Large-scale injection of BST into cattle would leave new punctures in their skin which could be a possible entry point for BSE infection; although such injections by law had to be made with a new hypodermic needle for each animal, the temptations for corner-cutting to a vet with 200 or more cattle to treat in a single herd would be enormous. Artificially boosting a cow's milk production could also weaken her resistance against disease and was likely to cause an increase in the common udder infection called mastitis.

The first point was conjecture but it seemed a sensible safeguard in a time of great confusion; the re-use of infected needles was already known to be a major cause of the spread of infection, demonstrated by the spread of the HIV virus amongst drug addicts in the human AIDS epidemic. Further, everyone on the committee knew that when a cow has a serious udder disease, infectious agents from her udders can pass into her milk. In my view it was not yet proven that should that animal be in the undetected early stages of BSE infection, there was no possibility of that infection going into her milk and therefore straight into the human food chain.

These were scientific debatables, the very sort of objection that I had been invited onto the committee to raise. It is significant, given that the committee was supposed to be independent and science-based, that I was the only person in the room to bring them into discussion

My intervention clearly angered Professor Armour, the chairman.

'You should not keep raising these speculative and highly controversial opinions without having some proof that they are true,' he said coldly.

'I disagree,' I fired back, for to be publicly rebuked for having made a reasonable scientific points angered me. 'Under the Medicines Act, it is the duty of the drug manufacturer to prove that his products have no serious side effects rather than for us to prove that they do. If you will excuse me, Mr Chairman, I feel this committee has got its priorities back to front.'

There was a rumble of discontent around the meeting and many hostile eyes turned in my direction. My objections to BST were overruled. The committee was not prepared to act to prevent the possible spread of BSE in humans.

I had a long and lonely journey back to Leeds that evening. There were many issues of national importance on which to ponder but also issues of great personal importance to me and my family. Having become the object of scorn and even hatred in the listeria and salmonella scandals, I had no real desire to undergo the process again. But I had no doubt that in BSE, we had a medical crisis looming which would far outweigh all the others put together in its dangers, and I was now convinced that the government and its advisers were not working to prevent that.

The cover-ups I had seen following the outbreaks of listeria, salmonella and E. coli were bad enough, but at least these bacteria were the causes of known infections with known methods of prevention and, in most cases, known methods of treatment, however unsatisfactory. In BSE and the related spongiform diseases, however, there was a new dimension that was, frankly, terrifying. It was possible that, already, hundreds or even thousands of people had been infected: the growth-hormone scandal seemed to point to the fact that an infectious CJD agent was already at work in the human population. Even worse, the incubation period in humans, if Sporadic CJD or Kuru were any indication, could be anything from ten to fifty years, meaning that Britain could face a plague of massive proportions at any time during the first three decades of the twenty-first century. And there was no known method of treatment. A cover-up in this case would be even more unacceptable.

This was a situation that demanded a crash research programme into CJD, which should be given top political priority and all the funding that such a programme demands. The key point in my musings as my train sped north to Leeds that evening was that if the government had already embarked on a cover-up, and if it was being advised by the likes of my Veterinary Products Committee, no such research programme would ever get off the ground. To set up such a programme would be to admit publicly that a major danger existed and that the government had done everything in its power to pretend otherwise.

In other words, untold numbers of people might be condemned to die in horrific circumstances at some indeterminate time in the future in order to save political reputations in the present.

The next question I had to consider was obvious: was there anyone in a position to tear away the veil of a possible BSE cover-up and force government action so that such vital research was allowed to begin? That person, I reflected, must have certain attributes: he must be a scientist of some standing with a background in disease spread via food; he must be prepared to speak out and therefore risk putting his career at stake; and he must have contacts in the media because, patently, the politicians and the civil servants were prepared to ignore scientific advice presented in secret and, therefore, easy to suppress.

I arrived home north of Leeds in the small hours of the morning knowing all too well that there were very few, if any, people in the United Kingdom who fitted all those categories. Except me. I discussed this with my wife Fionna. Both of us knew instinctively that, despite my so-called tenure at Leeds University, I would be hammering the final nail into my professional coffin should I choose to step onto this particular battlefield. But with heavy hearts, we agreed: to take the easy way out, the way of silence, would be to make a nonsense of my life's work.

Therefore I had to dissociate myself from the workings of the government. I sat down and wrote my letter of resignation from the Veterinary Products Committee.

Before I could speak out, I needed to do my homework. I was aware that, as a microbiologist involved primarily in human health care, I would in future come under attack by critics who would accuse me of knowing little about spongiform diseases in cattle. I knew that I would be pitted against government scientists whose job it would be to disprove any possible theory I might evolve, to ward off any research programme that I might be likely to recommend. So I buckled down to some of the most intensive study I had undertaken since my days as a medical student.

As I have remarked before, there is virtually no one alive capable of absorbing the torrent of all the medical and veterinary papers issued year in, year out, by the world's leading research centres: one year's publications would fill a good-sized room from floor to ceiling. Anyone pursuing a working career in a given speciality can, at best, keep more or less up-to-date with advances in his own field. Faced with BSE, the various forms of CJD and the workings of spongiform diseases within the brain, I began to cross back and forth between half a dozen different disciplines. But I refused to be defeated by the mountain of information to be absorbed. I was determined to be as well informed as anyone in the world who had not made a career in these diseases.

Battle was joined.

12

RIDICULE

It was a domestic cat, of all things, which finally let the BSE crisis out of the bag.

At the turn of the years 1989 and 1990, the government introduced several new measures in an attempt to allay public concern over the possible spread of the disease to humans. One of these included the removal of certain organs from cattle in slaughterhouses, so that they would not enter the human food chain. These included tissue from the brain, spleen, thymus, intestines and tonsils, and the spinal cord. It was, in my opinion, ludicrous to include the latter, because the total removal of all spinal cord tissue is a job which would challenge the skills of a highly qualified veterinary surgeon working in a fully equipped operating theatre, and even then, it would be a long and delicate procedure; it was therefore unreasonable to expect slaughtermen working under pressure to make a half-adequate job of such a task. The government was either totally naïve about the nature of the operation under abattoir conditions or it merely announced the measure as a placebo against public alarm. Or perhaps the truth was a bit of both.

A second measure was the announcement that farmers would be paid the full market price of an animal found to be suffering from BSE, instead of the 50 per cent first introduced. Margaret Thatcher herself approved the move, which was designed to stop the sale of cattle in the early stages of the disease. This failed, as the television programme *World in Action* was later to prove by smuggling hidden television cameras into auction rings and filming cows that were staggering and shaking, patently in the later stages of BSE, being sold without comment from any of the gathered farmers or auctioneers. Those cows were destined for slaughterhouses and, therefore, went straight into the human food chain.

And, although the farmers were delighted to receive their 100 per cent compensation payments, they too began to suspect that there was more afoot than was being publicly admitted. 'It was only then that we realized that there might be something seriously wrong from a non-farming point of view,' a senior NFU official said later.

Whilst these not-wholly-effective government moves were underway, I was working with a colleague in Leeds, Dr Stephen Dealler, to collate all known evidence about spongiform brain diseases in animals in an attempt to quantify the risk to humans. This work, set alongside studies of published work on Sporadic CJD and Kuru, led us to the grim estimate of a possible five per cent death rate amongst the population of the United Kingdom within the next 20 years or so. That estimate was published in an article in *Country Living* by James Erlichman, Consumer Affairs correspondent of the *Guardian*, on food safety, in which I cooperated.

The estimate was picked up and published by one of my local newspapers, the *Yorkshire Evening Post*, which had invited me to write a regular column on food safety. Chilling as the suggestion was, involving a possibility of more than two million deaths, it attracted little attention in the national media: perhaps they were beginning to believe the line being pushed by various unnamed government spokesmen that I was 'hysterical' and 'alarmist' (as reported in Hansard and various media reports). In Yorkshire, however, various butchers' organizations launched vociferous attacks on me, accusing me of putting thousands of jobs at risk. In April 1990, Humberside County Council decided, as a precautionary measure, to ban the serving of beef in school meals. This decision was received with outrage in Westminster, Whitehall, and amongst the various farming, food-processing and meat-production industries. Most other local authorities were reluctant to follow suit.

Then a cat died...

It happened in the West Country and the victim was a pet Siamese called Max which, in May 1990, died after a series of symptoms that were becoming very familiar by now: loss of muscular coordination, attacks of morose behaviour interspersed with mania, followed by coma and death. Laboratory tests showed that it had died from spongiform encephalopathy: a feline form of BSE. When the story became public, the press christened the dead Siamese 'Mad Max' and much was made of the fact that it had been fed on tinned cat food, and that cat food, being made of animal protein, could therefore be a source of BSE. Only in an animal-loving nation like Britain could the death of a pet cause such an outcry.

The significance of the death of Mad Max was not lost upon Stephen Dealler and myself in Leeds. Although much press comment had concentrated on the threat to millions of cats kept as pets in Britain, the most sinister aspect of this event was that BSE had jumped one more species barrier. The list of animals known to be naturally susceptible to Transmissible Spongiform Encephalopathies (TSEs) was growing: man, sheep, goats, mule deer, mountain elk, mink, nyala antelopes and now cats.

In Westminster, in response to the public alarm, the House of Commons Select Committee on Agriculture decided to stage its own inquiry, to which the media would be welcome, and at which I was due to be a much-criticized witness (as I shall describe in the next chapter). Even before I was called, I feared the enquiry would be a farce because it was probably intended as an exercise in public reassurance. Such an aim meant that any evidence that might alarm the public, whether it be of genuine scientific concern or not, would be targeted for public ridicule by those wanting to avoid such alarm.

In May 1990, I gave an interview to the *Sunday Times*, which was to make me the prime target for any politician, civil servant, scientist, food processor and farmer with a vested interest in proving that the BSE threat was, in fact, a mere 'scare'. This weasel word was much used by PR men to undermine any case with which they did not agree, for 'scare' suggests that there is nothing truly amiss, merely a small bunch of anti-government critics creating unnecessary alarm.

On May 13, 1990, the *Sunday Times* led its front page with the headline: 'LEADING FOOD SCIENTIST CALLS FOR SLAUGHTER OF 6M COWS'.

Of all the headlines relating to me in my career, effective or dismissive, supportive or destructive, these nine short words were to devastate my life. They were also, as I shall explain, to have repercussions on domestic politics and international relations, come close to bringing the British beef industry to its knees, and confuse and concern the British consumer.

Before detailing of the hysteria which was to follow amongst the higher echelons of the establishment, it is important to discuss the contents of that *Sunday Times* article.

I said what I said, not out of any desire to embarrass the government, but from closely thought-through scientific motives. As I saw it, I was merely doing my job as a servant employed to protect the public health and I saw, looming in the future, the spectre of the catastrophic spread of an incurable illness, which the NHS that employed me would have to deal with. To have remained silent would also have been to fail in my duty as a doctor who had taken the Hippocratic oath to prevent suffering, as a scientist whose career had been largely dedicated to food safety, and as a human being with normal concerns for friends and family.

The story ran:

The risks of humans catching 'mad cow' disease are now so great that 6m cattle need to be slaughtered, one of Britain's leading food scientists said yesterday.

Professor Richard Lacey, a former government health adviser, said people should not eat beef until half the herds in Britain, each of which had at least one infected cow, had been destroyed and beef had been proved safe to eat again ...

Lacey, professor of clinical microbiology at Leeds University, whose comments were described as alarmist by government scientists, called for a package of urgent safety measures ...

The proposals include a total ban on the £350m exports of British cattle and beef each year. 'We need to put the British Isles in quarantine ourselves before someone else does,' he says.

I knew full well that such a slaughter policy would be enormously costly: given a (low) average price of some £1,000 per animal, the scheme would cost around £20 billion, including the costs of disposing with old stock and replacing it with new. I was fully aware too that, for a few years at least, the British beef industry would have to undergo the most dramatic restructuring in agricultural history anywhere in the world.

To put those figures into perspective, however, £20 billion is the generally accepted estimate of the cost of the poll tax which Margaret

Thatcher unsuccessfully tried to foist on the British people. It is approximately three per cent of the nation's social welfare budget in 1998 which, of course, is an annual cost that will no doubt go on forever: a determined attack on BSE would have been a one-off burden on the tax-payer, painful to swallow but, like all nasty medicine, beneficial in the future. It is little in comparison with the actual eventual cost of the BSE shambles, budgeted at between £2 billion and £3 billion by the end of 1997 and still rising inexorably. It would have been a small price to pay had it prevented the worst-case scenario: if many thousands of people do become ill with CJD in the next 30 years or so, as I believe they are likely to, the costs to the nation will be in the hundreds of billions. The cost in human terms will be incalculable.

These, then, were the facts I wanted to be put before the British people, facts which I believe must have already been being discussed behind closed doors in Westminster and Whitehall. I have no doubt that the decision to take no action on a major slaughter policy in 1990 will turn out to be the biggest disaster, both in suffering and hard cash, that a British government has ever taken in peacetime.

Their answer: shoot the messenger. The attacks on my professional standing began in the very same article in a quote from Keith Meldrum, the newly appointed Government Chief Veterinary Officer. Meldrum's advisers, we now know, were already growing increasingly concerned at the possibility of the transmission of BSE to humans, but he chose not to share those concerns with the *Sunday Times*.

Instead, he accused me of 'pure supposition, over-reaction and scaremongering'.

'To suggest that the discovery of spongiform encephalopathy in a cat increases the risk to man is absolute nonsense,' he thundered, although nowhere in the article am I mentioned as referring to the incidence of feline TSE. He then went on to assure the public that beef was fit to eat because the agent which caused scrapie had not been detected in sheep muscle. This, in a roundabout way, was to say that because the scrapie agent was not found in sheep muscle, it would not be found in beef muscle, and therefore beef was wholesome.

The *Sunday Times* concluded its story with a quote from David Maclean, the then Food Minister, who said: 'Professor Lacey is good at popping up in the media with scare stories. Even the most elementary scientist knows that this disease cannot be passed from cow to cow like an infection.'

No one, of course, likes to be publicly insulted on the front page of a newspaper of international repute and it is tempting to respond with clichés: that the truth hurts, and this article had obviously wounded the government deeply; that I had touched a raw nerve; that I had become a thorn in the government's flesh. The important point to make, however, is that some of these remarks from both Meldrum and Maclean contained misleading scientific statements which were as yet far from proven and were coming under increasing attack from many expert sources, including some of the government's own advisers. If these two did not know this, they should have done. To me, their personal attacks bore all the marks of officials setting up yet another smoke screen to obscure, if not the truth – the truth was not known then and is still not in full detail today – but genuine scientific concerns.

Meldrum had described as 'nonsense' the possibility that an outbreak of feline TSE increased the risk to humans. To all serious-minded health professionals, the jumping from one species to another of a lethal infection is a matter of the highest possible concern, a danger sign to be ignored only at great peril. As the leading vet in the land, Meldrum must surely have been aware of this.

His second statement, that beef muscle could not contain a scrapie-like infectious agent because this does not happen in scrapie-infected sheep, was not proven. Virtually nothing was known in 1990 about the cause of BSE in cattle and to assume that because sheep scrapie did not infect man so BSE would not, was pure guesswork. And, as I have explained, already doubts were being expressed by scientists other than myself that scrapie was not in fact the source of BSE. To be so positive in a public statement when so many imponderables were involved was, it seemed to me, irresponsible.

In criticizing me for 'popping up in the media', Food Minister David Maclean appeared to be saying that unless something was proved to be dangerous, we should go on using it although the warning signs were obvious.

To say that 'even the most elementary scientist' knew that BSE could not be passed from cow to cow was not only, in its implication, personally offensive, but untrue. In 1990, with the known long incubation period of the disease, it was too early to know if BSE could be passed vertically from cow to calf. Moreover, it was well known that scrapie could be transmitted from ewe to lamb. Any government adviser insisting that BSE was a bovine equivalent of scrapie, as many still were, should have suspected the worst and taken measures to avoid it.

Whether or not Maclean knew this statement was untrue I cannot say. I would prefer to give him the benefit of the doubt. But he should most certainly have been better advised.

Sunday 13 May 1990 was quite a day in the life of the Lacey family. The fact that my wife and daughters read insults about me was made worse by the fact that the phone rang constantly as the media pack raced to follow up the *Sunday Times* story. I was particularly concerned about my daughters, who had to go to school the following day and face schoolmates who, no doubt, would also know what the newspapers were saying about their famous professor father. But if I thought the ridicule would stop there, I was deluding myself.

During the week following the publication of the *Sunday Times* article, a group of Conservative MPs filed what is known as an early day motion in the House of Commons. It read:

That this house condemns the relentless attack on British farmers and food producers by professors who display symptoms akin to BSE and calls on the Department of Health to investigate the mental state of Professor Lacey who, having helped destroy the egg industry, is now turning his attention to beef.

This was, of course, a calculated smear disguised in a cloak of adolescent humour, the sort of joshing that I had been subjected to at my prep school many years before, from politicians elected to protect the rights and the wellbeing of millions of British subjects. Although presented as a joke, the underlying thrust was clear: I was now to be treated as the Mad Professor, as the *Yorkshire Post*, for instance, described me.

Insult aside, this resolution gives a clear indication of the lack of foresight and concern amongst elected representatives about the health of their constituents. Their concerns were in protecting the rights of farmers and the food industry, even though these might, however unwittingly, be poisoning their customers. The thrust was that BSE was to be made into a joke, a method used by court jesters of old to deflect attention from serious truths. Try as I might, and thankfully I have a sense of humour which helped me survive the coming months without actually becoming the Mad Professor, I could see absolutely nothing to laugh about as the crisis in the countryside became worse by the day.

For me, there were also unpleasant undertones to this event. An early day motion is only a device to attract media attention. Such motions are never debated in the House because they are never given the necessary parliamentary time. Because of this, they never have a chance of becoming law. They are, however, a method by which MPs can let off steam and allow their various prejudices to be reported in the newspapers and particularly by the Press Association. The PA is a national news agency, supplying news to all the British press and broadcasting media, from Fleet Street down to the local evening and weekly newspapers throughout the country. Backbench MPs who rarely find themselves quoted in the national press hope that the PA will pick up anything they say, or any motion they propose, and it will be reported in their local newspaper back home.

As most people know, most important debates in Parliament take place in the afternoons or, quite regularly, late at night, when regional evening newspapers have been long printed and distributed. So the early day motion, which as the name suggests is posted before the day's parliamentary work actually begins, is a boon for PA reporters covering Parliament, whose duty it is to supply the regional papers with copy. So that morning in May 1990, the wires began to buzz with a story about the Mad Professor.

Now there may well be readers who will say that, in this, I had been hoist by my own petard. I had, I freely admit, begun to use the media to bring my worries about BSE to the attention of the general public. The MPs who launched this attack may well have believed they were paying me back in my own coin. But there are major differences between an MP and a private member of the public exploiting the media.

Firstly, MPs already have a platform from which to express their views: that, after all, is why they are elected to Parliament in the first place. Secondly, anything said or written on a motion paper within the Palace of Westminster in such a media debate is given the protection of parliamentary privilege: this means that an outsider attacked from the floor of the House cannot take legal action for libel or slander. This rule was introduced for the very best democratic reasons, to allow MPs to speak out on affairs of public importance without fear of legal retribution, a situation that I would heartily support under the vast majority of circumstances: it is essential that our legislators are not gagged from speaking what they consider to be important truths. This, however, presupposes that MPs use this legal protection frugally and only after much careful thought. To use it to attack a man's sanity for the simple reason that you dislike what he says is, to me, a misuse of parliamentary power.

Had someone accused me of madness outside the Palace of Westminster, I would have sued, as I had already done successfully in other cases. As it was, all I could do was sit back and accept the ridicule.

Like most major universities, Leeds has its own internal newspaper. Called the *Leeds Reporter*, it contains the usual mix of departmental gossip, promotions and retirements and, from time to time in grand old academic tradition, pungent letters on matters of controversy. The backbiting, back-stabbing and sheer petulance that arise in disputes between academics have been the subject many novels and plays. To keep some semblance of intelligent respectability in some of these disputes, the *Reporter* does have a general rule of conduct: if one academic is about to launch an attack on a colleague's ideas or theories, it is customary to show the person under attack the letter or article involved before publication, to give him or her the right of reply.

After giving evidence to the House of Commons Select Committee on BSE (of which more in the next chapter), I was away from Leeds briefly in July 1990 at a conference, when a letter appeared in the *Reporter* from nine members of the Department of Animal Physiology and Nutrition, a department which has a gathering of vets and animal-feed experts and which receives some of its research funding from MAFF and some of the major animal foodstuffs companies. It was, in all the attempts ever made to discredit me, the most savage stab in the back that I ever sustained. It appeared without my prior consultation, which I believe to be unique, and at a time when I was away and therefore unable to defend myself. It is, I think, worth quoting in full:

> The statements recently made on the subject of Bovine Spongiform Encephalopathy (BSE) by Professor Lacey to the House of Commons Select Committee on Agriculture and elsewhere have been the cause of considerable embarrassment to us as agricultural scientists and as members of the University of Leeds.

> Whilst we would not in any way wish to question Professor Lacey's right either way to speak as a Professor of the University of Leeds within his speciality of Clinical Microbiology or to speak as an interested individual in areas outside his speciality, we are concerned at his apparent reluctance to make the distinction himself, and with his failure to ensure that the media observe this distinction in describing him.

> We are also concerned at the contrast between the cautious and scientifically correct approach taken by Professor Lacey when communicating with other scientists in, for example, articles in *The Lancet* or presentations to departmental seminars, and the simplistic and alarmist nature of many of his public statements.

> In controversial or politically sensitive matters in which putative risks to public health and safety are opposed to economic necessity and commercial interest, it is particularly important that the scientific enquiry necessary for a rational resolution of the problem remains within the scientific arena. Complex technical evidence must be evaluated by argument among those competent to do so before conclusions are broadcast.

> As a result of Professor Lacey's high public profile, and his pronouncements as a professor of the University of Leeds on matters outside his immediate area of expertise, we now find ourselves spending a considerable amount of time defending the University from hostile comments made by people in the scientific

community, in agriculture and from among the general public, who associate the University with his views.

Until now, we have avoided explicit critical comment because of the effect on the University of a controversy among its members becoming public. We now consider, however, that the adverse effect of Professor Lacey's publicised statements on the University's reputation is such that we must call on him to ensure that any publicly expressed views of his that are outside his area of expertise in Clinical Microbiology are explicitly stated as personal.

We also invite him to consider the harmful effect which popular publication of untested results and hypotheses could have on the future conduct of scientific discourse.

The allegations of this letter are understated but quite clear. I was talking about things I knew nothing about; I was bringing the university into disrepute; I was acting unprofessionally as a scientist; I was alarmist, and simplistic; I was also, it seems, pretty thick – I could not understand 'complex technical evidence' as I was not among those 'competent'. Worst of all – and I believe this is the clause which reveals the true motive behind the letter – I was putting 'putative' risks to the public before commercial and political concerns.

They could hardly have been more insulting towards my professional standing, something that every scientist and academic protects jealously. The fact that, with my colleague Stephen Dealler, I was about to publish the first ever scientific paper detailing the real threat of BSE to human beings – which was not known to them – disproves their suggestion that I knew nothing about the subject. Months of joint research had gone into that paper, drawing together strands of evidence from all the important research ever done anywhere in the world in the fields of transmissible spongiform diseases in both animals and human beings.

The academic arguments I could comfortably refute, but the truly puzzling problem in this attack was the underlying reason behind it. I had, I agree, most certainly alarmed some of the people who funded the Department of Animal Physiology and Nutrition research and I could not expect their thanks for that. Nor was I prepared to make any apologies for this, for I thought it had been necessary to stir up public interest in order to ensure that critically needed research should go ahead.

But what was most baffling in this incident is that I heard of the existence of this letter two days before its publication, not from the editor of the *Reporter*, as was the custom, but from a staff journalist at the Press Association. Now outside the media and the world of politics, few people are even aware of the existence of PA. As it does not produce publications in its own right, but only prepares copy for other newspapers, the general public have no point of contact with the organization. This applies equally to most academics. Yet here, somehow, an as-yet-unpublished letter to an obscure, regional university newspaper had fallen into the hands of the national news agency. And it was, of course, a good story: even his own colleagues were turning against the Mad Professor, discrediting him professionally. The consequences were immediate, in the form of attacks on me in the *Daily Mail* and the Yorkshire Television news programme, *Calendar*.

It seemed that someone, somewhere – at the time, I assumed that it was officials from MAFF – was doing a highly skilled demolition job on my reputation.

13

STAR CHAMBER

Although I was subject to ridicule and attack for my public statements, I was not the only person who doubted the government line. Within ten days of the death of Mad Max, the pet Siamese, which caused public concern that humans could become infected with BSE, beef sales in Britain had plummeted by 25 per cent. Other local authorities followed Humberside in banning British beef from their school meals. The 29,000 strong American forces in Britain had already taken the same action, which represented the loss of another large market for farmers and butchers. But the biggest blow was about to fall – a blow that finally spurred the government into a frenzy of action.

First France, then Germany and Italy, banned the import of British beef, an act that many people, and in particular British farmers, considered to be in breach of European Union treaties. To the Thatcher government, whose attitude towards Europe was, to say the least, ambivalent, it seemed an act of treachery, and ministers began to accuse our European partners of taking this action, not because of health fears, but as a stick with which to beat the British farmer; in effect, of using BSE to protect their own farming interests. There was a major, and very difficult, crisis meeting in Brussels, which lasted for 26 hours and eventually reached a compromise: British beef could remain on sale only if accompanied by a certificate signed by a vet proving that the meat came from a herd free of BSE.

The British delegation, led by the new Agriculture Minister, John Gummer, agreed this compromise without consulting their own veterinary advisers. When they returned home claiming a triumph, to their surprise they ran into a heated behind-the-scenes row: in a rare show of professional defiance, the veterinary advisers pointed out that to sign such a certificate was beyond their scientific remit. Until the appearance of the final and fatal symptoms in cattle – the staggering, the apparent mania – they had no way of knowing whether or not a herd was free of BSE. So another compromise was reached: beef bound for mainland Europe would be accompanied by a certificate showing it came from a herd that had not suffered a case of BSE in the previous two years.

Even this was paring professional ethics down to the bone, because all vets knew that the incubation period of BSE was likely to be at least two years and possibly a great deal longer. This meant that the certification procedure was at best optimistic and at worst totally worthless. However, much to my surprise, the Europeans accepted the proposal – for a couple of years, at least.

The initial ban created huge political controversy. Of the little and belated action that the government had taken to prevent the spread of BSE since the first notified (as opposed to filed and forgotten) outbreaks in 1986, nothing seemed to be working. The figures of BSE cases were rising inexorably – almost 15,000 new cases were reported in 1990 alone. What little research that had been done had taken MAFF and the Department of Health no closer to a solution and, despite public assurances to the contrary, the Mad Max incident had caused widespread alarm amongst their scientific advisers. For the first time, it began to sink in at the highest reaches of government that a major crisis was underway.

The government began to react in two separate ways. The Spongiform Encephalopathy Advisory Committee (SEAC) under Dr David Tyrrell became involved in the generation of reassuring statements, in addition to its formal terms of reference to assess priorities in research. The CJD Surveillance Unit, a new research unit based in Edinburgh, was formed to watch for any danger signs to human health. This was to become important later in the continuing problem, but its creation was not subject to any major publicity: as a result the first human death from the new-variant CJD that was to develop from Sporadic CJD was not even reported to it, because the neurologist involved in the treatment did not know of its existence.

Having gone some way to taking the action which should have come four years earlier, politicians began to consider ways of deflecting attention from their earlier tardiness. They decided, I believe, that they needed scapegoats. Their first target would be the double-dealing Europeans, who were presented as banning the Roast Beef of Olde England apparently as a health measure but in fact to bolster the interests of their own peasant farmers. This display of xenophobia sadly proved to be extremely popular with the British electorate and still hampers our relationships with the EU. The campaign reached such a pitch of fury that one Minister, Nicholas Ridley, launched an attack on the Germans so fierce that he was forced to resign.

Whilst the European attacks were underway, the troops at home were also being marshalled. SEAC chairman David Tyrrell issued a press statement which said: 'There is no danger in eating British beef.' Only in 1998, in the BBC2 television series *Mad Cows and Englishmen*, did the laborious chain of distortion associated with that statement become public. The programme revealed that, under considerable pressure from MAFF to issue a positive statement, Tyrrell and his colleagues sat down to deliberate. Finally, they created a draft statement which said that eating British beef was not dangerous when compared to other daily activities, like crossing the road. This was not considered strong enough, so a second draft said that, on present evidence, there was no danger in eating British beef. That, too, was considered too wishy-washy. Eventually, the final statement, the one released to the Press, said simply: BRITISH BEEF IS SAFE. As Tyrrell himself admits today, that was not what the SEAC committee intended. Once again, scientific fact had been overridden in the interests of MAFF policy.

Although I was unaware of these deliberations, I was aware from the science grapevine that there was growing unrest amongst government scientific advisers at the way their work was being distorted to support political aims. And as the leading critic of these aims, I was to become the domestic scapegoat.

The Star Chamber was created in Tudor times as a popular arena for the settling of small legal differences. In Stuart times, it was corrupted by Charles I to become a secret court, where opponents of the regime were tried and sentenced for crimes they had not committed. Their only offence tended to be their opposition to the King and his noble advisers. The chamber has passed into notoriety as a symbol of oppression, and repugnance for its excesses led to the creation of what is regarded by many as the finest legal system in the world. In 1990, when I attended the House of Commons Select Committee on Agriculture, I wondered whether the Star Chamber had indeed been abolished or whether I was in fact facing its successor.

The Select Committee inquiry, staged in response to growing public alarm over BSE following the death of Mad Max, was headed by the Conservative MP Jerry Wiggin, a landowner with large farming interests; another member, also a Tory, was Christopher Gill, another farmer with interests in a meat-processing company. When I duly received a summons to appear before this committee, and was given just two or three days to write my submission of evidence so that the committee would have time to prepare questions to put to me, I knew that I was in for a rough ride. I decided that attack would be the best form of defence.

That written submission was leaked to the press and reports appeared in the newspapers on the morning of my appearance, 13 June. *The Times* led its story with a headline which read: 'MINISTERS ACCUSED OF FAILING TO COMBAT BSE THREAT TO HUMANS'. It then quoted long passages from my submission: that 'much of the hope that BSE will not pass to man has now evaporated' and the only response from ministers in a 'crisis of major magnitude' seemed to be the 'parrot-like claim that our beef is completely safe'. These strong words were merely skirmishing before what I intended to be the main thrust of my attack. What most concerned me was that, by taking no action in the human health field, the government was proposing to 'permit a gigantic long term experiment to see how many of us acquire a fatal infection that should have been entirely avoidable'. Even worse, should man be attacked by this disease, that disease might become vertically transmissible in the human population: that is, passed on from mother to baby.

The Times noted that I was careful to state that 'Men may or may not be vulnerable because there is no data on which to make the prediction' and published a list of safety measures which I thought should be brought into force just in case. These included a total ban on animal protein in any animal foodstuffs and a widespread slaughter policy in infected herds, including all calves born into those herds.

I knew that such reports would have done little to endear me to the committee. However, I went into the Houses of Parliament happy to justify all these concerns in front of the televised proceedings. Some of the points, I considered, were of immense scientific importance. I was, for a start, expressing my doubts that BSE had in fact come from sheep scrapie, which was still the government line. I was also raising for the first time in public my concerns about the possibility of vertical transmission in cattle and, should man become infected, in humans too.

These were concerns of enormous significance to both human and animal health. At that time no scientist anywhere in the world had any answers to the question they raised. But if cows were passing BSE onto their calves, the beef and dairy industries in this country were doomed unless a complete new start was made. If BSE had not in fact come from scrapie and were to spread to humans, and could be passed down from mother to baby – as spongiform disease had had been shown to do in Kuru – the potential consequences were almost unthinkable.

As this was a committee of MPs, I hoped that there might be at least one or two members who might take seriously their role as protectors of the public interest: after all, what could be more important than trying to keep British people and their babies alive? However, as soon as I sat down, I realized that I had been deluding myself. From its line of questioning the committee appeared to have no interest whatsoever in discussing scientific theorizing, however nightmarish, and seemed to focus solely on attacking me. It was as if I was back in the Star Chamber of Charles I.

Jerry Wiggin began by pouring scorn on almost every aspect of my submission. Then he handed over to Christopher Gill, who accused me of being an alarmist. Another member had, to his jubilation, discovered that my secretary had made a single typing error in my submission, which is hardly surprising considering the speed at which it had been prepared. I was pressed time and time again on this minor error (in quoting the Southwood report's statement that sheep was included in material for rendering, I had written 'sheep heads'). I was accused of unnecessarily alarming the public, of being unqualified, of putting British farming at risk, of being a publicity seeker. It appeared that they had one job in mind: destroy Lacey.

By this time, I had become quite practised in defending myself in television debates, with perhaps one or two adversaries in the debate and a skilled journalist in the chair to prevent the debate becoming mired in turgid repetition. This, however, was the first time I had been grilled with monotonous repetition by a committee that was totally hostile, and a chairman even more hostile than most of the members.

Try as I could, no one would listen to my key point: that although there was no proof that BSE would pass to humans, we should be taking precautions just in case. The attitude of the House of Commons Select Committee on Agriculture, which, presumably, should represent the very peak of thought and planning in the farming world, was exactly that of the Veterinary Products Committee: prove that something is dangerous, rather than have the producer prove that it is safe. Once again, this time in the most public arena possible, these men, who were elected to protect the interests of the British people, were quite openly and without any apparent concern sidelining the public in favour of commercial interests – interests which, indeed, some of them shared.

I made a major error. Frustrated that no one seemed the slightest bit interested in discussing the potential dangers to human health – the ostensible reason for my presence as a witness – I lost my temper. Harried by Wiggin and Gill to set some sort of figures on the fatality rate which my worst-case scenario could create, I barked: 'If our worst fears are realized, we could virtually lose a generation of people. If the worst comes to the worst – and I sincerely hope it won't.'

As soon as I had said it, I knew that I had done what they wanted me to do. My interrogators sat back with self-satisfied smirks. This, everyone in that committee room knew, would be the sound-bite shown on television. Here was the Mad Professor going completely over the top with a doom-and-gloom pronouncement so extreme as to be almost laughable. Under pressure, I had made a statement that, compared with my view at the time of what was likely, based on the figures of the mortality rates in animal spongiform disease, of a human fatality rate of up to five per cent, made an already alarming scenario look like a science-fiction nightmare. Yet, in science fact, this was still a possibility as a worst-case scenario, evidenced by the fact that in the North American mink outbreaks years before (detailed in chapter nine), entire populations had died after the disease struck.

Anyone who watched those few seconds of film, without having seen the badgering and hectoring that led up to my statement, might have justifiably thought that here indeed was a Mad Professor. As a result my credibility, in political eyes at least, had suffered a reversal.

A mere three weeks later, the committee issued its report. It came as no surprise to me that it concluded that British beef was perfectly safe and that any misgivings I might have could be safely ignored.

A few days later, John Gummer rose triumphantly in the House of Commons to announce: 'British beef can continue to be eaten safely by everyone, adults and children.' Then he went on to attack the media for 'alarmist reporting' of the BSE affair.

Sadly for Gummer, he and other government ministers had misjudged the mood of the British public and, indeed, world opinion. Sales of beef continued to fall, more countries abroad banned British beef, and the numbers of BSE cases continued to soar. The *Independent on Sunday* had already published the results of an opinion poll it had commissioned from one of the leading pollsters, NOP, which showed that a quarter of the British public did not believe the government statements. More than half believed beef should not be served to children, and 31 per cent of women said they would stop eating it themselves – a significant figure as, by and large, women do most of the food shopping in Britain. The figure amongst men who would stop eating beef was lower, at 22 per cent, but this still represented a large portion of the potential beef market.

That market was hit again during the summer, when a major fast-food chain, Burger King, announced it was banning British beef from its outlets. And commenting on the *Independent* opinion poll figures, the Opposition spokesman on food and agriculture, Dr David Clark, accused MAFF of 'lies and cover-up'.

I might have been made to look foolish, but it seemed that, when it came to placing their trust either in the views of their government or in those of the man that government was trying to smear as the Mad Professor, a large section of the public chose me. That may sound boastful but it is not meant as such. If my efforts helped to persuade thousands of people to give up eating beef at a time when some of it was riddled with a killer infection, my public humiliation was worthwhile, for it is very likely that some of those people escaped a disease which, unknown to the scientists, was already beginning to replicate in the central nervous systems of some unfortunate youngsters.

*

After such a deluge of bad publicity, I expected some form of positive action from the government, including the extension of the slaughter policy to calves in infected herds and a total ban on animal proteins in all animal feeds (the earlier ban had applied only to feeds to ruminants). Most of all, if tens of millions could be spent to compensate farmers, I hoped to see funds devoted to a large-scale, high-profile research programme to, first, actually isolate the still-unknown agent responsible for the spread of spongiform diseases and, most critical of all, discover a medical testing procedure that would show if human beings were infected well before the final, fatal symptoms began to appear.

This has still not been achieved. The CJD Surveillance Unit in Edinburgh was beginning to do some important work but it was, in comparison with the size of the problem, merely scratching at the surface. Moreover, all its findings (I was sent copies of their confidential reports) were being kept as closely guarded secrets, which would do little to assuage public concern. I know it would have been very expensive, but had an earlier start been made on a research programme, adequately funded and employing the best brains in the world, we might by now be in a position to at least check humans for infection. Even politicians as obdurate as the Thatcher government would, I believed, see the necessity for this as one of the country's most important industries crashed to its knees. I was wrong.

Instead, the government decided to brazen it out. The thrust of official policy was, publicly, that no crisis existed because there was no danger to humans. Privately, the government was exerting almost unbearable pressure on various research bodies to come up with some concrete scientific answers and, preferably, ones that would assuage public concern forever. As one member of the underfunded and understaffed CJD Unit in Edinburgh was to admit years later, they could barely get on with their real work because, day in and day out, they had to spend hours on the telephone trying to answer unanswerable questions from panicking civil servants in Whitehall.

Ministers' public stance of almost casual confidence led to what I consider to be a most distasteful publicity stunt. Attending an agricultural show with his family, John Gummer was surrounded by a mob of television cameramen and press photographers outside a stall selling hamburgers. In view of the BSE scare, would he be prepared to allow his four-year-old daughter, Cordelia, to eat a burger? Of course, said Gummer confidently, and so this little girl was duly served with a burger – which is, anyway, one of the most unhealthy items of twentieth-century diet. The chances that it was infected by BSE were minimal but existed nevertheless. Even if it were not infected with BSE, burgers had already been proved beyond doubt to be one of the classic carriers of salmonella and other well-known food-borne diseases, as well as a major cause of obesity in the young, and a Minister of the Crown should have rejected this proposition in the interests of healthy eating.

Cordelia, as it happened, showed more sense than her father. As the television cameras whirred and the press cameramen clicked away, the little girl in the summer dress took one bite at the burger, complained that it was too hot, handed it to her dad and ran away. Gummer, looking a little flummoxed, ate the burger himself whilst giving an informal press conference on the benefits of British beef.

The incident was one of the leading sound-bites on television news that evening and I watched it with revulsion. Health grounds apart, for a minister to use his own daughter in a cheap publicity stunt was, to me, both degrading for the girl and humiliating for the man.

What we did not know, until the BBC2 documentary *Mad Cows and Englishmen* revealed the truth in 1998, was that Gummer had been ambushed. The *Sun* newspaper, known for the craftiness of its journalistic wiles, had contacted the minister a few days before and suggested to him: would he let Cordelia eat a burger in front of the cameras? Gummer, an astute publicist, realized that he was trapped: had he said no, The *Sun* could have run a headline saying something like: 'AGRICULTURE MINISTER BANS DAUGHTER'S BURGER'. That, as he explained in the documentary, would have been disastrous to his campaign to persuade the country that beef was safe, so he felt he had no alternative but to go ahead.

This episode, I believe, says something about the judgement of the man who was the key government figure in the handling of the BSE crisis. He would surely have been within his rights to say, 'I will eat the burger myself but I will not involve my family.' Even the *Sun* would have understood that.

*

Newspaper and television reports were dominated by stories about BSE throughout the summer of 1990. Then, in September, *Today* newspaper reported a new development, its front-page headline reading: 'MAD SOW DISEASE'. BSE had jumped another species: Porcine Spongiform Encephalopathy had developed in a pig injected with diseased tissue from a cow infected by BSE. In the same month, a similar disease had found its way by natural transmission into zoo animals, an eland and a kudu. The disease was still marching on, despite all government efforts to control it.

Government officials tried to emphasize that since the pig had been infected artificially by government vets, as had happened to certain other laboratory animals in the research into Kuru and the outbreak of mink TSE in North America many years before, the experimental spread was by no means as significant or as serious as an infection transmitted by natural means. This, to an extent, was perfectly true: no animal under normal circumstances is likely to receive a dose of infection as concentrated as in an injection direct into the brain.

However, what was not emphasized at the time, and was particularly significant, was the fact that, in its physiology, the pig is much closer to human beings than many other animals. The immune systems between the two are particularly close, a circumstance which has allowed humans to be fitted with pig-heart transplants which are not rejected by the human defence mechanisms. Because of these similarities, an occurrence of PSE was another sinister step closer to the result we all feared most: human infection.

For farmers, too, the PSE case represented another deep anxiety. Offal from sheep and cattle had been banned from feed for those animals two years earlier, but its use had been allowed to continue in pig and poultry feeds, as well as in canned food for domestic pets. The case of Mad Max had heavily implicated pet food as the source of the cat's spongiform disease. It didn't take much to put two and together and come up with the alarming possibility that a spongiform disease might soon appear in the country's pig herds or poultry flocks, an outbreak which, coming on top of BSE, would amount to financial disaster for many farmers and, indeed, a massive dent in the country's ability to feed itself.

The government responded by banning cattle offal from pig and poultry feed. Thankfully, a TSE has not emerged in either pigs or poultry under natural conditions (if, of course, one can call modern farming methods for both these animal 'natural').

The number of BSE cases continued to rise (from 7,136 in 1989 to 14,180 in 1991, then 25,025 in 1991 and 35,045 in 1992) at a time when, if infected animal protein in the feed were the sole source of infection, they should have been beginning to fall off as a result of the 1988 ban. The alternative, the doomsday scenario to MAFF, was that the disease was being spread in a new way, either vertically from mother to calf or, potentially even worse, laterally from one cow to another within a herd. Such hypotheses would have necessitated the huge slaughter policy that I had proposed in the *Sunday Times* interview. That, of course, was a possibility that the politicians did not want to admit, so their scientists searched round in desperation for a more acceptable alternative.

The discovery that farmers had been feeding left-over poultry and pig food, then containing cattle offal, to cattle for the two years after the cattle feed ban came like a godsend. Here was the source of the continued growth in BSE cases. And it was careless farmers, not the government, who were to blame. That, one of the many red herrings floated in a decade of red herrings, was one of the most damaging of them all. Not only was it patent nonsense – it may have contributed to the further spread of BSE, but the incidents were not numerous enough to be realistically judged by any sensible person to be responsible for the huge increases in BSE cases – but it was accepted as the cause of the rising figures and put a stop to further inquiry. This created a set-back to what little research the government was actually doing.

Meanwhile, Stephen Dealler and I had finished our major effort in the search for that truth, our collation of all the known, published scientific evidence of TSEs in both animals and man. It appeared in the technical journal *Food Microbiology* in December 1990. It was the longest scientific treatise I have been associated with, running into 26 pages of small type, six of which were simply devoted to listing the hundreds of scientific documents and reports we had collated in months of research. It was called: 'Transmissible spongiform encephalopathies: The threat of BSE to man'.

To summarize the findings: it made public for the first time our doubts that BSE was being spread from sheep scrapie and infected feed. That meant, we argued, that there must be other routes for its spread from animal to animal, such as vertical or lateral transmission, the very subject that MAFF were so determined to ignore. We pointed out that, in cattle, the infection attacked between one and ten per cent of animals in a given herd. If the disease were to spread to humans as a CJD-like illness, 'the high prevalence of infected animals must represent a phenomenal danger to man'.

I have rarely written anything more 'alarmist' (as my colleagues at Leeds University who had attacked me might have described it) than the sentence I have just quoted. It was a professional view based on scientific research, and it was proved to be right.

Conscious that any hypothesis ventured would be scrutinized and any inconsistencies attacked, we had made sure that it was a tightly worded and scientifically correct presentation. It was written in technical terms which were unlikely to be comprehensible to anyone but a trained scientist. This, I believe, is why it was overlooked by most science journalists and virtually all political pundits. Stephen and I personally paid for 5,000 copies to be printed and distributed to a wide range of influential people, including many MPs and even Prince Charles. I hope it was studied by the government's scientific advisers, for they received copies too.

Publicly, however, even though it was a scientifically correct paper that was the most detailed assessment of the BSE risk ever to be published, no one took any notice. The paper disappeared virtually without trace.

14

CONSPIRACY OF SILENCE?

The difference between cover-up and conspiracy is difficult to pinpoint with great accuracy.

The former can, I suppose, be deemed to be understandable in any human activity: when something has gone terribly wrong, no one likes to see his or her mistakes publicly exposed. The initial reaction is to cover up any mistakes – be they from incompetence, tardiness, pressure from above, or simply false hopes – and hope that, with a bit of luck, the situation will simply go away. All these had come into play during the first five years of the BSE crisis. Although I do not condone it, I can understand why politicians and their civil servants were anxious to cover up the errors that had been made: public confidence had already been badly shaken and to admit to them would have been to exacerbate an already delicate situation.

To impose a conspiracy of silence is, in my mind, another matter. This suggests to me a cynical decision to withhold information for fear of the political consequences. In the case of public health, this is morally wrong, for it robs members of the public of the opportunity to make choices which would protect their own health – in this case, to stop eating British beef until it was proved safe rather than vice versa. But it also had a most dangerous effect on the scientists working extremely hard with limited resources to solve one of the greatest medical and veterinary crises of the age. This danger is simply stated: as I have already illustrated, scientists may feel pressurized into coming up with findings that support current political thinking rather than the actual facts.

From years of studying various government and civil service pronouncements, it is my belief that the events of 1992 and early 1993 amounted to conspiracy.

In September 1991, the Ministry of Agriculture officially forecast that the number of new cases of BSE would begin to decline within a year. This pronouncement was taken with a large pinch of salt by many members of the scientific and farming communities because in 1989, the Southwood committee had forecast a total death toll of between 17,000 and 20,000 cattle before the disease finally petered out due to the ban on animal protein in cattle feed; yet the actual figure had reached the 50,000 mark by the end of 1991 and had jumped from 25,025 cases in 1991 to 35,045 in 1992 when the disease was supposed to be dying out.

The total of deaths was now four times the original estimate and was still climbing rapidly. Even in MAFF, it must have been realized that something had gone terribly wrong. The unavoidable suspicion to any scientist, however pressurized from above, must have been that the disease was now being spread from some source other than infected feed. But to admit the next possibility – that the infection must be being transmitted within herds, either vertically from mother to calf or horizontally from animal to animal – would immediately illustrate that measures taken in the previous five years had been ineffective, if not actually useless. It would predicate that all young cattle born since the feed ban of 1988 were also at risk, which would undoubtedly renew calls for a slaughter campaign even more widespread than the six million cull I recommended in my *Sunday Times* interview in 1990.

To make matters even worse, these dark musings were underway at a time when the country was in deep recession: millions of people were losing their jobs, hundreds of thousands were losing both their homes and life savings, thanks to negative equity, and tens of thousands of small businesses were going into bankruptcy. Once again, the cost of unemployment benefit was rising and reduced spending was causing a drop in tax revenue. The possibility of having to spend tens of billions to compensate farmers for slaughtered BSE herds at such a time might well have had the mandarins at the treasury standing on their balconies contemplating suicide.

Whilst these grave considerations were being discussed secretly in political, scientific and farming circles, BSE largely dropped off the front pages for two or three years in the early 1990s: in the depths of recession, the British public had more immediate concerns. One of the things they did not know was that, in 1988 and 1989, government vets had conducted a top-secret series of trials to test the possibility of vertical transmission of BSE from cow to calf. Three hundred calves from BSE mothers had been reared in conditions that ensured they never ate contaminated foodstuffs. By March, 1991, not a single calf had become infected, a finding which no doubt brought joy in the corridors of MAFF. But two years later, *New Scientist* reported that two of the calves had contracted the disease.

What *New Scientist* did not know then, for details were meagre and carefully guarded, was that 42 calves from BSE-infected mothers would eventually contract the disease. Even more significantly, another group of 300 calves from non-BSE mothers reared in the same conditions produced 13 calves which became infected. These are, from a scientific viewpoint, truly alarming figures: the vertical transmission rate from BSE mothers was over ten per cent and from apparently healthy mothers almost five per cent. In others words, almost one in twenty healthy cows could carry the disease without showing any symptoms and pass it on to their offspring.

Extrapolate those figures into the British national herd of some 10 million cattle and even the figure of some 80,000 infected animals looked like a hopeless underestimate: the eventual figure could run into the millions. These were figures that, if released, would have provoked extreme public concern and a national crisis for our farming industry, and another, even more severe, international confrontation with our European partners who were still allowing the sale of British beef certified as coming from herds free of BSE for a mere two years.

It was, to judge from my personal experience, these findings which led to the conspiracy of silence.

Since my mauling by the House of Commons Select Committee on Agriculture in 1990, I had for two years kept with my colleague Dr Stephen Dealler a relatively low profile in the BSE crisis, helped by the fact that the media were showing little interest in the story at this time. By 1993 Stephen had left my department to become a clinical microbiologist at York General Hospital, but we had continued with our collation of any known scientific material on BSE. We were by now both convinced that things were going very wrong indeed. We decided we would express our concerns via official channels, and therefore sought a meeting with Dr David Tyrrell, chairman of the government's key advisers on the Spongiform Encephalopathy Advisory Committee (SEAC).

We drew up a 16-point discussion paper. Many of the points related to our concerns about the scientific methodology being used in the meagre results of government research that had been published in the technical media. For instance, some results were based on experiments involving the injection of tiny volumes of BSE into mice, which are short-lived animals highly resistant to BSE, and their survival in no way guarantees safety for human consumption. We were concerned about the apparent lack of research on vertical or lateral transmission of the disease within cattle herds – the damning experimental results had not yet been made public. We believed one omission in government policy to be a major miscalculation: the fact that, six years after the first official reports of BSE, with its proven lethality to cattle and its potential threat to humans, CJD had not been made a notifiable disease. We were also deeply concerned that, although cattle bones and skins had been banned from animal food chains, they were still being rendered into gelatin, a substance widely used in the human food industry in items such as sweets and pork pies. This was all the more disturbing because gelatin is widely used in the drug industry in capsules for medicines, and the Department of Health had instructed pharmaceutical companies not to make gelatin from BSE-infected herds as early as 1989. If it was considered dangerous in capsules, it should have been considered dangerous in food; it was not banned until the end of 1997. Nine years is an inexcusably long period over which to take such an important decision.

It took a long time to arrange that 'informal' meeting with Tyrrell. Eventually, under a cloak of considerable secrecy – there were no attendants, secretaries or observers – it took place in June 1993 at the National Agricultural Centre at Stoneleigh, near Warwick, roughly half-way between Yorkshire and Whitehall.

Our reception was frosty, and our points barely discussed in detail. Instead, Tyrrell and his party of government vets and civil servants who attended the meeting seemed more concerned with us not making our private disquiet public. Three hours of talks achieved, as far as Stephen and I were concerned, no concrete results, not even an agreement that our points would be studied in more detail later.

That alone was dispiriting, for in a scientific debate on matters of the gravest national importance new ideas should be welcomed and explored. Worse, though, was the distinct impression I gained that Tyrrell and his colleagues were acting as though they knew we had discovered that the information was not being provided – indeed John Wilesmith, the vet in charge of BSE research, was so nervous that he was visibly shaking.

This is only speculation, for I cannot speak for Tyrrell, but I can only assume that he was already aware of the recent experimental results showing vertical transmission from cow to calf. To give him the benefit of the doubt, this information may not have been passed to him as it should have been, and as chairman of the government's key advisory committee he should have made sure that it was. Dealing with Stephen and me he was, I admit, in a very difficult situation: had he admitted that the points we made were valid, his committee would have had to state that the whole basis of their advice was flawed. But he could at least have given us some assurance that our genuine concerns would be thoroughly investigated.

That so-called 'informal' meeting in June 1993, was to have unexpected repercussions as I was writing this book early in 1998. Having been summoned to appear before the new government's BSE enquiry, I received by fax a curious piece of correspondence from the Central Veterinary Laboratory at Weybridge in Surrey. With it came the official minutes agreed by Tyrrell of the 1993 meeting, and a scribbled note saying that 'this report has not been disclosed to the public'.

The mere facts that there were minutes of an 'informal' meeting surprised me. No one that day had been visibly taking notes and yet, according to my recollection, the minutes seem to be surprisingly accurate. The only conclusion I can draw from this is that the discussions were secretly tape-recorded which, to say the least, shows a lack of courtesy: we could at least have been warned that we were on tape.

Those minutes had been circulated 'in confidence' at the time, to people at the meeting and three others in MAFF; they were not sent to Stephen and myself. Having read them, I can now see that, from the government point of view, the meeting was allowed to proceed as an opportunity to find out what Stephen and I were thinking at the time, and whether we had any plans to publish those thoughts. Nothing we had to say on the science involved was acted on at the time.

It would not be the last time my views were to be sought by such methods.

In that same month of June 1993, when Stephen Dealler and I had our abortive meeting with David Tyrrell, the science-fiction aspects of the 'March of the Prions' took an enormous leap towards becoming science fact. It had taken 21 years to prove.

Since 1982, a distinguished American scientist had found himself in a situation remarkably akin to that of the hero of the science-fiction film, *Invasion of the Body Snatchers*, in which the only man to escape the giant pods from outer space was a doctor who, having learned the truth, was taken straight to a psychiatric hospital when he tries to warn others that the aliens have taken control of most of the population of a small American town by taking over human bodies.

This scientist was Dr Stanley Prusiner, who in the late 1970s and early 1980s had studied the outbreaks of TSE on American mink farms (outlined in chapter nine), caused by an infectious agent unknown to the science of the time. It was, as readers will remember, Prusiner who first coined the word 'prion'. He had postulated that it was a tiny particle of protein which could somehow take over an animal's central nervous system by 'burying' itself in individual brain cells, where it began to eat away the neuron cells. Because it was hidden within the cell, it was invisible to the animal's immune defence mechanisms and was allowed to grow unchallenged. Finally, it would eat away so many cells that the brain would begin to resemble a sponge. This was the disease he had witnessed in mink.

Prusiner's ideas were scoffed at by much of the American scientific establishment. His critics attacked his theories because they contradicted existing scientific knowledge about the behaviour of viruses, the assumption being that the disease must be spread by some form of undetectable virus: no one could conceive that an entirely new, or rather unknown, organism was at work. To support their case, the critics pointed out that to successfully invade a new host, viruses needed either their own DNA or its close collaborator RNA. After an attack, remains of these DNA and RNA deposits could be isolated and therefore establish the presence of the virus. As neither viral DNA nor RNA remains had been isolated in the dead mink, *ipso facto* there could be no virus.

This reasoning overlooked the fact that the very basis of Prusiner's theory was that, precisely because there were no traces of viral infection, some other agent must be at work. The row in the American scientific establishment that ensued was to last for more than 20 years.

Then in June 1993, a Swiss scientist called Dr Weissman, working with a group of colleagues in Zürich, made a breakthrough. Unlike Prusiner, these scientists had in their laboratory a new set of scientific tools, the tools of the new science of genetic engineering, which allow researchers to remove a single gene or set of genes from an animal's DNA. They set about using these tools to test the prion theory in one of those ideas which are so simple that they shine with brilliance: they began to remove genes from laboratory mice which were then injected with tissue infected with the spongiform infection best known to man, sheep scrapie. Whilst most mice in the experiment became infected with scrapie, some which had had certain genes removed remained immune. This could only mean one thing. The prion, or a part of it known as PrP, could only replicate in a mouse's brain if a certain gene were present in its DNA. Without it, PrP died.

The conclusion was, therefore, that the prion, or PrP, instead of carrying its own DNA and RNA, was using the host's own DNA to replicate. It was, to misquote our film title, the *Invasion of the DNA Snatchers*. And, like the physical evidence of giant pods that proves the hero's sanity in the final frame of the film, it confirmed Prusiner's theory against the scorn of his detractors.

This follows on to another conclusion. By incorporating some of its host's DNA into its own reproductive system, the prion must mutate in character. The resulting micro-organism, because it is using different DNA to replicate, will also be different – just as DNA from sheep is different from that of a mouse. It is, to use a crude analogy, the progeny of two different parents, half prion, half host. This means, in effect, that when it is reproduced it becomes a different type of creature, according to what host it is within, whether it be a sheep, a cow, a mink... or a human being. In other words, when a spongiform disease crosses yet another species barrier, the infection in the new host is an entirely new form of disease caused by a newly mutated prion.

The significance of this in the case of BSE is enormous. It means that even if it is true, which I doubt, that BSE in cattle did come from sheep scrapie originally, it would be a different organism by the time it had adapted to cattle. But for many years, there had been a rare cattle disease known colloquially as 'the staggers', which caused cows to lose their physical coordination. I suspect that it was this infection, largely ignored by vets because it was so rare, that, spreading by the method I have just described, became modern BSE when cows were first forced into cannibalism by being fed the rendered remains of their own species. This, after all, is what happened in the New Guinea Kuru outbreak, although, as I have said, no research has been done on this yet. Sporadic CJD in European humans may well have also originated not from scrapie but from 'the staggers'. Indeed, I did present the idea to the BSE inquiry in March 1998 that a rare disease in cattle had been the historical cause of Sporadic CJD, including those cattle farmers succumbing, and BSE was a new variant or mutation from the old staggers, which had been spread initially by cannibalism and then by animal-to-animal means.

The importance of the Zürich research was that there was now no need to account for the absence of DNA in the infectious particle, and it explained how the infectious agent kept changing as it passed from one species to another, since each host had its own characteristic DNA. This meant that even if scrapie in sheep had caused BSE, the nature of the infective particle would be different after being in cattle to that in sheep. So there was a formal dismissal of the claim that because sheep scrapie does not cause CJD, BSE cannot. In 1994 American researchers in Montana showed that sheep scrapie injected into calves did not cause BSE. The vital new Zürich evidence was at last a promising avenue for research. With the existence of the prion established in all but the most reactionary of scientific minds, the search to isolate it and then to kill it to prevent the terrible disease it spreads should have been launched immediately.

These findings were published in *Cell*, a highly prestigious international journal necessarily read by MAFF scientists. But in the United Kingdom nothing happened. Although cattle were still dying in their tens of thousands, no one thought it worthwhile to identify and eradicate the reason why. For some young human beings, it was already too late.

That breakthrough year of 1993 was also the beginning of the end of my career as a university professor. For more than five years, I had been aware of the sound of knives being sharpened in certain dark corners of the health establishment. That summer, one of them was stabbed between my shoulder blades.

In 1991, huge reforms of the NHS had been put through Parliament, and local health trusts had been formed. These reforms meant my dual role as a university professor, with its valuable protection of tenure, and NHS consultant was becoming increasingly difficult. Important work began to be diverted from my department to other branches of the NHS. I was, for instance, chairman of the Leeds General Infirmary Control of Infectious Diseases Committee, a role in which I had as much experience as any consultant in the NHS. But when the committee met, I discovered that important decisions in this field had been taken elsewhere and implemented without my knowledge.

Then, later in the year, one of the senior officials of the Leeds NHS Trust came to see me. An important press release was to be issued that very afternoon saying that my department was to be merged with the local Public Health Service Laboratory and, once the merger was complete, there would be no need for my future services. I was 53 years old, in what many people might consider to be their prime, supporting daughters aged nine and eighteen. My wife Fionna and I had long suspected that this sort of situation would arise after my resignation from the Veterinary Products Committee and my outspokenness in the BSE campaign, but the callous brutality of the presentation of this news took me completely unawares.

For a start, although suspicious, I had never been given any concrete evidence that I was to be removed from my post. It had never been discussed in any way face to face. But if a press statement was to be issued within a matter of hours, the matter had obviously been discussed at length behind closed doors and the action approved at the highest level. Even the press office were aware of the situation long before me.

The merger with the Public Health Laboratory Service was totally unexpected but I saw instantly the significance of this move. As I have said before, this service is a fine organization in which good scientists do sterling work in the prevention of the spread of infectious diseases, but the scientists employed by this agency do not have the right to publish scientific findings without the written permission of the Department of

Health. Within my own experience, that permission is often refused. Nor do these scientists have the luxury of tenure. It was to scientists working under these conditions that my role was to be handed over. A gag was being put in place.

I had been outmanoeuvred but not beaten. If they thought that I would go quietly, they were deluding themselves. If my record had proved anything, it had proved that I was not easily deterred by threats, from however high a source they might come. I decided to fight back.

In a bureaucratic battle that was to last well into 1994, Leeds University offered me great support, despite the fact that some of my own scientific colleagues had earlier joined the ranks of those against me. With government funding cuts and ever-more intrusive government interference into the very heart of campus life, they had few weapons with which to fight. Without NHS funding, which represented 60 per cent of the Department of Clinical Microbiology, the university could not hope to keep the department open without making swingeing cuts in the resources of other academic activities.

The bureaucrats continued to use devious and underhand methods to force me out. In 1993, for instance, I was in Pakistan giving a lecture to an international conference on infectious disease control, for my standing in the world scientific community was high (and still is: I believe that I have done something like 100 lecture tours in some 40 countries, and the invitations to do more arrive every week).

In a move that reminded me of the Kremlin in Soviet times, when leaders were almost invariably ousted when they were out of the country on foreign visits, a senior NHS official went to my department, called my staff together and told them that I was no longer in charge. In future, he said, they were to take no instructions from me and any findings they made in public-health matters should be reported to another department. My staff, God bless 'em, told him where to go in no uncertain terms and continued to work for me until the day of my final departure.

After almost two years of haggling, I finally agreed to take early retirement from the university at an enhanced pension. Additionally, on leaving the university, I was to be given a three-year contract to run the microbiology unit at Chapel Allerton Hospital in North Leeds, a small, 300-bed unit which caters mainly for geriatric patients and has no acute medicine facilities which call for the level of skills to which I have trained.

Whilst I have the greatest respect for Chapel Allerton and its staff, this was an inappropriate position for me. To the bureaucrats, no doubt, it was a triumph: they thought that they had finally pulled the painful thorn from their side. But those most wronged were the British tax-payers, for at Chapel Allerton, my daily duties for three years rarely occupied me for more than 20 minutes in the morning. So in my spare time I dug ever deeper into the BSE cover-up, building on evidence I had published in my book, *Mad Cow Disease*. Their ruse to force me into silence had not only failed but it also backfired against the Leeds Hospital Trust budget which, some years later, was to become the most overspent in the British Isles. I estimate that, at a time when entire hospital wards were being closed down, thousands of serious operations being postponed, and the purchase advanced medical technology being rationed, the cost to the NHS of the attack against me – in, for instance, legal costs, pension arrangements and wasted salary – reached something like £500,000. As I write this, I am now officially unemployed (although I must emphasize, not collecting the dole).

To say the least, this is a curious use of scarce public resources. Even more curious was the fact that, within days of my agreeing to take early retirement, the decision to amalgamate my department with the Public Health Laboratory Service was rescinded.

The authorities in the health service may have taken away my job and curtailed my career at its peak but someone, somewhere, was still anxious to keep track of my activities. I am not able to prove that my telephone was ever tapped – although many calls seemed to have a faint echo and occasional strange clicking sounds in the background – but around this time, someone began to tamper with my mail.

I had begun to research my book *Mad Cow Disease*, which was a blow-by-blow refutation, for general readers, of that Southwood Committee finding that BSE would stop in cattle and not jump to other species. This prediction had already been proved untrue by the spread to domestic cats, to pigs and mice under experimental conditions, and to ostriches in a German zoo, greater kudu antelopes in London zoo, and big cats like a cheetah and a puma in other zoos. Although discreet meetings had been held with our European partners to discuss this continuing spread, the public were kept uninformed. The object of my book was to reverse that situation. But first, of course, I had to find a publisher.

At first, several major London publishers showed great interest in the subject, but when the point arrived when contracts needed to be signed, they backed away. Saddened but undeterred, I finally came to an agreement with a small publisher based in South Wales. I will not name the publisher, nor his company, for reasons that will become apparent – he and his family have already suffered enough.

Having accepted the book, the publisher began to receive phone calls from people who did not identify themselves by name but merely asked 'Is it true that you are doing a book on BSE?' or 'Are you publishing a book by that Professor Lacey?' Asking why the caller wanted to know, he would receive replies like, 'I'm very interested and would like to buy a copy as soon as it is out.' A publisher's job is, of course, to sell books so in his innocence, he said yes.

The publisher lives in a nice country house outside the small town where his office is based, in an area of rolling countryside surrounded by dairy and beef farms. They, like all their kind in the United Kingdom, were suffering large financial losses because of the BSE scandal. A few nights later, the publisher received a call from a local farmer who warned him to publish the book at his peril.

Then a large stone was thrown through his window, thoroughly shaking his wife.

This began to worry the publisher, whose home was isolated and therefore an easy target for attack. Had I any idea, he asked me in a state of some anxiety, who could have tipped off the local farming community about the impending publication? He himself, for obvious reasons, had not mentioned it to anyone in the immediate locality of his home.

At that point, I had no idea. But then letters from him to me and vice versa, enclosing large sections of the manuscript, began to arrive stamped with a Royal Mail message which stated the envelope had been damaged in transit and had been opened and re-sealed. Now this had happened to me perhaps once or twice in a lifetime. For it to happen with regularity in correspondence between two recurring addresses must be more than a coincidence.

And as tampering with the Royal Mail is a criminal offence, who else, I thought, could have the authority to do so with impunity except the security forces, either the Special Branch or MI5?

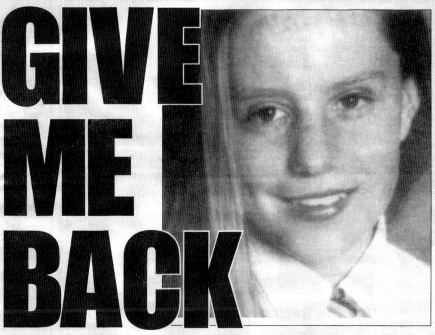

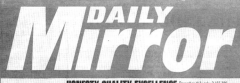
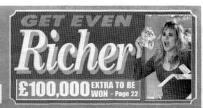

Tuesday, January 25, 1994 HONESTY, QUALITY, EXCELLENCE December daily sale: 3,165,735 (INCORPORATING THE DAILY RECORD) 27p

GET EVEN Richer
£100,000 EXTRA TO BE WON - Page 22

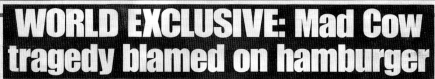

WORLD EXCLUSIVE: Mad Cow tragedy blamed on hamburger

GIVE ME BACK MY LIFE

By ANTON ANTONOWICZ

THIS is Mad Cow victim Vicky Rimmer – whose plight could be a fatal time bomb.

Vicky, 16 – who is blind and unable to talk, move or eat – may be the first known person to have caught the disease from a contaminated burger.

She is now fighting for life on a drip feed. Her last message to the world, scrawled on a calendar, was: "I want my life back."

Yesterday, her heartbroken mother Beryl declared: "I'm convinced she got the disease from a burger.

"She's never been ill in her life. She was the healthiest child on earth. But she's always loved meat." If Beryl's

■ Turn to Page 7

THEY BEGGED ME TO HUSH IT UP - MOTHER'S AGONY Page 7

How the *Daily Mirror* broke the news of 'Mad Cow' victim Vicky Rimmer in 1994 (see page 159).

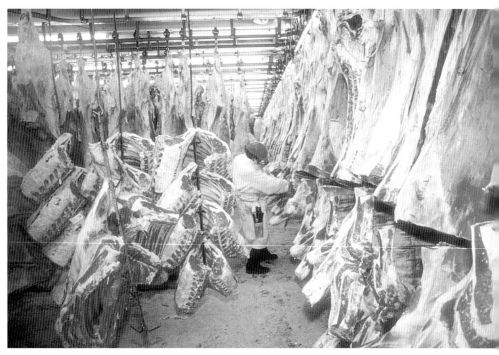

Poor hygiene in some British abattoirs led to microbial contamination between carcasses.
(Peter Menzel/Science Photo Library)

Examination of a cow showing uncoordinated movements characteristic of BSE (bovine
spongiform encephalopathy). (C.V.L./Eurelios/Science Photo Library)

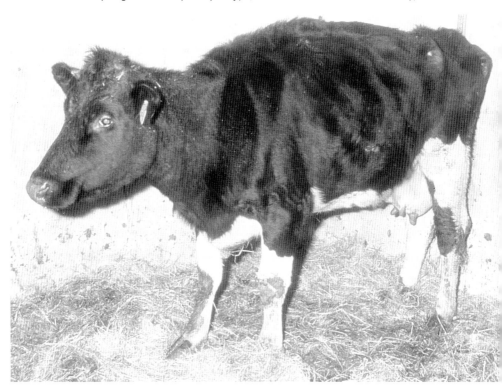

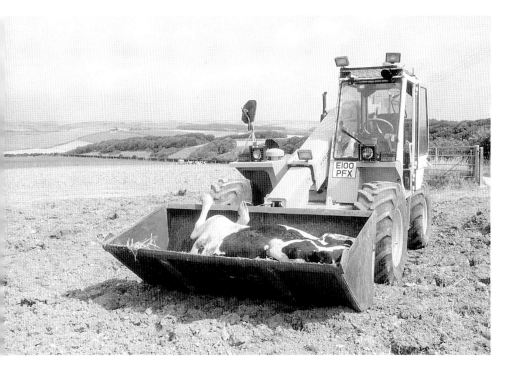

The carcass of a BSE-infected cow being moved by a JCB, ready for incineration. (Sinclair Stammers/ Science Photo Library)

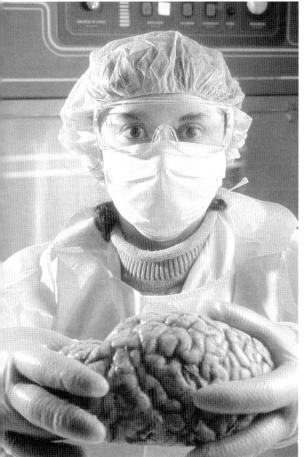

Left: A masked pathologist holds a human brain to be tested for Creutzfeldt-Jakob disease; it is now clear that BSE in cattle can cause this disease in humans, despite years of government denials. (Hubert Raguet/ Eurelios/ Science Photo Library)

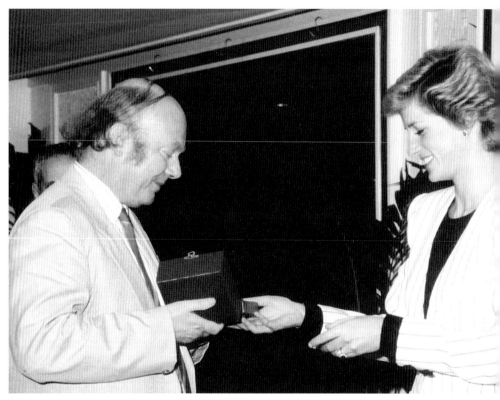

Receiving the 1989 Evian Health Award for Medicine and Service from the Princess of Wales; the citation was 'for his work in raising the profile of the whole problem of safe eating'.

In a field with cows in 1994, at the height of the BSE scandal. (Ross Parry Picture Agency)

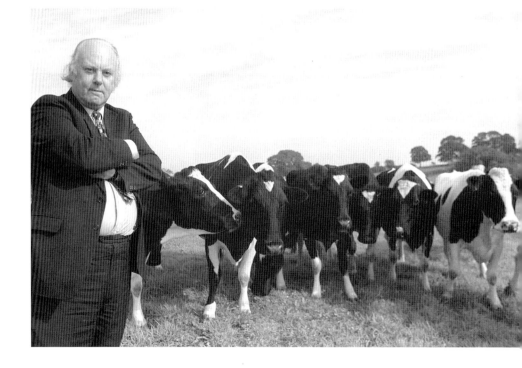

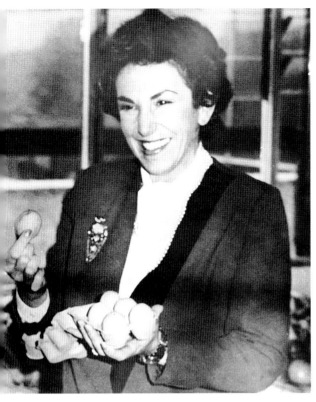

Left: Edwina Currie, the minister who was forced to resign for telling the truth about salmonella in eggs (see page 59).
(G. Hoban/PA News)

Below: The notorious stunt by John Gummer, Minister of Agriculture, when he attempted to force-feed his daughter with a burger to demonstrate how safe British beef was. She sensibly declined the offer.
(Jim James/PA News)

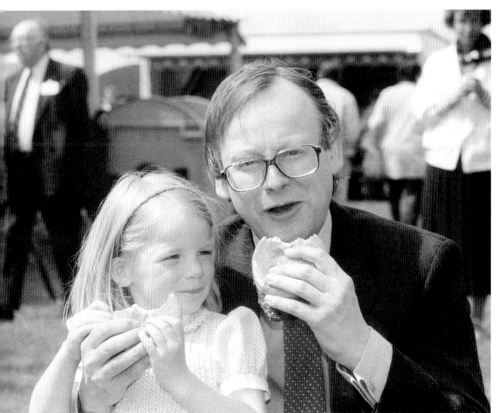

20 March 1996.
The government finally
admits that BSE in
cattle could cause
Creutzfeldt-Jakob
disease in humans.
(*Daily Mirror*)

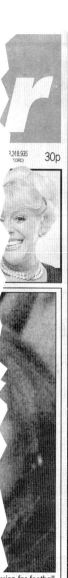

30p

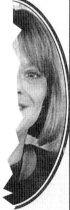

ssion for football

"bitter and angry"

OFFICIAL
MAD COW CAN KILL YOU

Govt to admit it today

By KEVIN MAGUIRE

EXCLUSIVE

HUMANS could catch Mad Cow Disease from eating infected beef, the government will admit today.

Health Secretary Stephen Dorrell will accept for the first time that the brain wasting disease may have been passed to people from infected animals.

The U-turn by Ministers — who for 10 years have insisted it was impossible — will spark calls for tough new curbs on suspect meat. But some experts fear we may already have eaten more than a **MILLION** infected animals — and that unsuspecting victims are living on borrowed time.

In a bid to prevent panic and a devastating effect on the food industry, Whitehall is launching a huge advertising campaign with the message that beef is not dangerous.

● Full story — Page 2

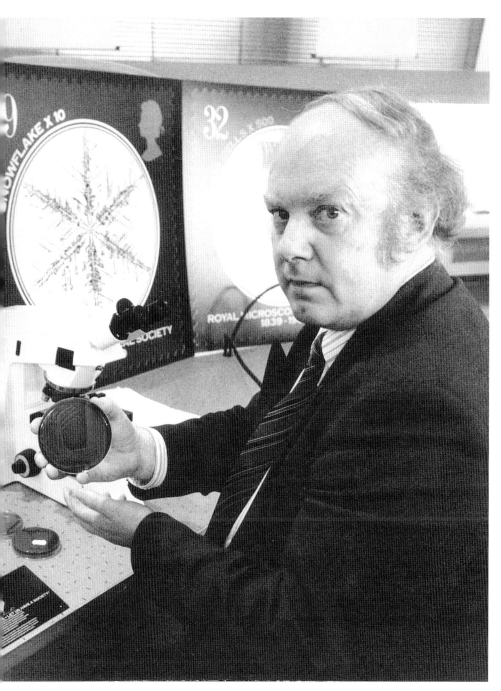

At the Science Museum in 1989 promoting new postage stamps with a scientific theme.
(Press Association/Topham)

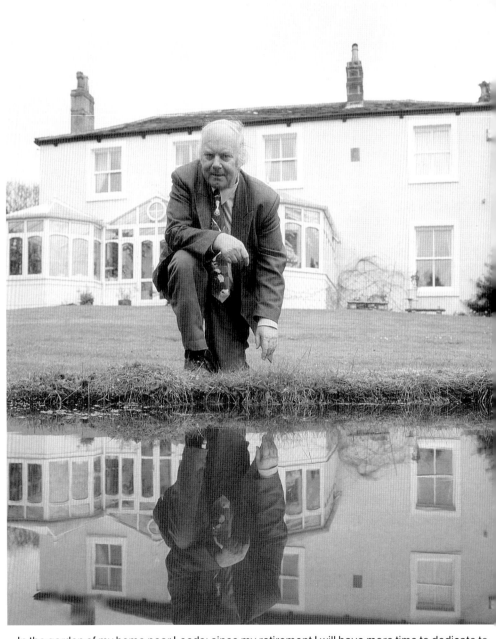

In the garden of my home near Leeds; since my retirement I will have more time to dedicate to our large and wild garden. (James King-Holmes)

I began to suspect myself of paranoia. After reflection, I came to the conclusion that had the security forces been interested in reading my manuscript before publication, they would surely have more sophisticated methods than merely tearing open an envelope and then resealing it with an official stamp. My supposition was that they had read the manuscript but wanted neither the publisher nor myself to know that this had happened, and therefore used 'damaged in transit' to disguise the fact.

Thinking of the threatening phone call to my publisher and the stone through his window, I concluded – though I cannot prove – that what was underway here was not quest for knowledge of my book's content – the government were already privy to most of that information, although they had decided to cover it up – but a warning to the publisher and myself: don't publish or else!

My stance on this was, to quote the Duke of Wellington's famous phrase, 'Publish and be damned.' The publisher, however, was unaccustomed to such threats and, concerned for his family's safety, decided he could not go ahead under his own imprint. He did agree to set up a 'shell' company in the Channel Islands under the unknown imprint of Cypsela. The book would be published in 1994.

All the efforts to silence me were a waste of time, though. They were too late: events had overtaken them. The first young people were beginning to die from a new variant of CJD.

15

PANIC

By 1993, unbeknownst to me and most other members of the scientific community, the CJD Surveillance Unit in Edinburgh was becoming increasingly concerned at worrying signs coming from the countryside. The information began as a trickle which was soon to become a steady stream, but at first it was often confusing. In October 1993, the Unit presented its third annual report to the Department of Health. In this they identified the dietary habits of 109 Sporadic CJD victims who were 13 times more likely to have been regular consumers of veal than people dying of other diseases. At a press conference, a spokesperson for the Department of Health described this finding as 'a statistical freak'. More and more, however, the Edinburgh staff were beginning to think the unthinkable: BSE might be passing into man.

In Lancashire, a farmer whose cattle herd had been infected with BSE died from CJD. His death was quickly followed by that of another farmer and postmortem examinations confirmed the CJD prognosis. As both men were over 50 years of age, it seemed that they had contracted Sporadic CJD which, although rare, had been known for most of the century. As several more farmers became affected – as I write in 1998, seven farmers have now died of the disease – statistics showed that this condition, which once affected only one in a million members of the population, was becoming more prevalent. It had increased tenfold in the previous quarter of a century and doubled in the previous five years.

Then in January 1994, I received a phone call from an anxious mother in North Wales. Her 16-year-old daughter had been ill for a year with a disease which seemed to be CJD. This was the first of many phone calls I was to receive over the next few years from parents suffering a similar ordeal. Beryl Rimmer, who lived in a village just outside Wrexham, was at her wits' end. Her teenage daughter, Vicky, was on a life-support machine in Wrexham and the doctors did not seem able to offer any help. Beryl had read of my activities in the newspapers and contacted me as a last resort. Could I give her any advice?

The dreadful fact of the matter was that, apart from some comfort, there was nothing that either I or medical science could offer. Despite seven years having passed since the first outbreak of BSE, no one was any nearer to identifying the disease in *cattle* before the final appearance of Mad Cow symptoms, never mind finding a cure. When it came to detecting or treating the disease in *humans*, there was not only a total lack of knowledge but also a complete lack of ideas: no one, as far as I am aware, had seriously considered the possibility of such a situation ever occurring.

I did, however, make the long drive to Wrexham to see Mrs Rimmer, a widow still suffering from the loss of her husband, to offer her whatever support I could. When I arrived, young Vicky was already in a deep coma and I discovered that the hospital authorities had conducted a brain biopsy (which means taking a small section of brain tissue from the patient for microscopic examination). This procedure, which is carried out, for obvious reasons, in only the most critical of cases, had proved that Vicky had a form of CJD. Just what form that was is still a matter of debate.

To the medical establishment, it would have been very convenient if poor Vicky Rimmer suffered from the known Sporadic CJD, but this was extremely unlikely. Sporadic CJD, rare as it is, was known mainly to strike at people aged 50 or above – most of its previous victims had been in their sixties or seventies – presumably because of its long incubation period of up to 30 years, perhaps even more. I was not aware of any previous case involving a teenager.

These considerations were no doubt high in the priorities of the doctor from the CJD Surveillance Unit, who came down from Edinburgh to examine Vicky and interview her mother. This conversation had alarmed her so much that she had contacted me. After a long discussion detailing step by step the progress of the disease over the previous year the doctor had thanked her and left her with a strange request: 'Please don't go to the newspapers about Vicky's illness. Think of the British economy and our relations with Europe.'

This was an outrageous remark from a senior Department of Health scientist whose job, allegedly, was to protect the public from the spread of a new and dangerous disease. Mrs Rimmer, with whom I was to speak many times over the ensuing years, was left with the indelible impression that the doctor from Edinburgh was far more interested in preventing any adverse publicity than in helping her daughter.

The case of Vicky Rimmer was, at the time, unique. As such, it should have been given the most serious attention using the best brains and resources of the NHS. Instead, when the news of her illness became public in a *Dispatches* television programme on Channel 4 a few weeks later, the Department of Health reaction followed up with what it seemed to me had now become the normal dismissive pattern.

The Department of Health issued a press release saying that it was untrue to suggest that Vicky had contracted a new, human form of BSE, because BSE could be proved only by a postmortem examination. And as poor Vicky was still alive, although comatose, this case could not be proved.

Not only did this statement show a cynical disregard for Beryl Rimmer's feelings – the suggestion was that nothing could be done until her unfortunate daughter was dead – it also revealed that the Department of Health was in a state of either total muddle or out-and-out mendacity. The people who drew up that press statement should have known about the brain biopsy which had conclusively pointed to the presence of CJD. If they did not, they were guilty of gross incompetence. If they did, and chose to ignore it, they were lying.

Once again, a public dismissal was to deflect attention from a case of crucial importance.

Although at that time there were no other examples of a BSE-like disease in human teenagers – a situation which, sadly, was not to last for much longer – having studied the case in great detail, I suspect that Vicky Rimmer's illness represented an important interim step in the development of CJD. Some of her symptoms were, in fact, very similar to those in long-known cases of Sporadic CJD but, as was to be discovered later, slightly different from cases of the new-variant disease soon to attack 27 more young people.

These differences, which included new-variant CJD having early difficulties in movement followed by later dementia (with Sporadic CJD the dementia precedes the disorders of movement), made Vicky's case of unique scientific interest because it suggested the possibility that, when it first attacked the young girl, the disease was still in the process of mutating to becoming new-variant CJD, as we now know it. This, I admit, is only a hypothesis, but one that would have been worth researching. Vicky Rimmer may have represented a vital 'missing link' in our understanding of the progress of the disease and as such, tragic though her case was, she should have been a research subject of the greatest significance.

It did not happen, although Vicky was to remain alive on a life-support machine in her north Wales home until the autumn of 1997. Beryl, her loving and self-sacrificing mother, insisted on this in the hope that someone, somewhere, would come up with a cure. She telephoned me again at that time and asked me if I thought there could be any hope. In what is perhaps the saddest sentence I have ever uttered, I said that I could not honestly see the possibility of any cure in the foreseeable future. Beryl, broken-hearted, ordered the life-support machine to be switched off.

If government ministers thought that the BSE crisis would simply go away in 1994 they were mistaken. In January, the *Daily Mirror* took up the Vicky Rimmer case and splashed the story over the front page under a headline which read: 'WORLD EXCLUSIVE: MAD COW TRAGEDY BLAMED ON HAMBURGER'. The paper carried a picture of blonde-haired, blue-eyed Vicky before she was taken ill, and its main headline quoted a little note she had scrawled on a calendar in her bedroom before she lost the ability to write. It said simply: 'GIVE ME BACK MY LIFE'. The *Mirror* story sparked off another round of speculation, met by denial from the various government departments involved.

Then, in autumn, my book *Mad Cow Disease* appeared. The book was serialized at length by the *Mail on Sunday*. For the first time, the British public was given a blow-by-blow account of the conspiracy of silence which had clouded the real threats of BSE to the human population. But not many people had a chance to read it for, after publication, senior government scientists gave the long interview to *The Times* attacking my reputation. Booksellers then began to cancel their orders. Once again, the Whitehall smear machine was in action. In a long interview with *The Times*, Keith Meldrum, the Chief Veterinary Officer, and John Wilesmith, the vet in charge of the government research programme, accused me of 'irresponsibility' and 'getting my facts wrong'.

Wilesmith declared 'We have nothing to hide.' And Meldrum, dismissing my prediction that BSE would spread to humans, made a rash promise which was also to be swept under the carpet as events unfolded: if I were right, he said, MAFF 'would consider the destruction of every cow in Britain'.

They went on to rehearse all the old arguments about cattle having caught the disease by eating scrapie-infected sheep remains and said that vertical transmission from mother to calf could not have been responsible for maintaining the rate of BSE at the then current levels. They re-introduced the red herring about farmers ignoring the ban on ruminant feeds for cattle that I mentioned earlier with a new twist: ruminant-free cattle feed had been cross-infected in the processing plants from chicken and pig feed which, until 1990, had still been permitted to be manufactured from cattle and sheep remains.

Apart from the debatability of all these arguments, as I have explained, the last assertion was very revealing. Given the fact that BSE takes between three and five years to incubate in cattle, these experts had added another two years to the anticipated life-span of the outbreak: from 1988, when ruminant feeds were banned in cattle, to 1990, thanks to careless farmers and cross-infection.

This smacked of a deliberate policy of playing for time as infections continued to rise amongst the national cattle herd long after they were supposed to decline. More importantly, government scientists already had in hand the results of tests on their 600-head experimental herds, which had been proved to be passing on the disease through vertical transmission. Were internal communications between the people heading the government research and advisory programmes so inadequate that Meldrum and Wilesmith were unaware of these results? The alternative, once again, was that the government was choosing to ignore their own scientists if their conclusions did not fit with political expediency.

In 1995, family doctors, then staff at local hospitals across the country were beginning to tend young people falling ill with a disease the likes of which had never seen before. Some of the victims were teenagers, the oldest a Liverpool mother aged 40. The symptoms started mildly and looked at first like an early form of arthritis: the victims began to lose interest in their daily routine, neglecting their dress and appearance, and falling out with or ignoring their friends and relatives. Then, within a matter of months, their behaviour became distinctly odd.

First, they began to lose their balance, finding it difficult to perform simple tasks like walking up and down stairs. In Liverpool, Anne Richardson, the 40-year-old mother, began to take falls in a most unnatural way: she made no attempt to put up her arms to protect herself and, as a result, often suffered facial cuts and bruising. When husband Ronnie called in the doctors, they said that Anne was in depression and her behaviour was designed to attract attention. When her fall injuries began to get worse, they even accused Ronnie of abusing his wife. Only when one of the doctors saw one of Anne's falls did the local medical service begin to realize that something here was seriously amiss.

In Wiltshire, a teenager called Stephen Churchill began to lose interest in his normally highly active social life. Then he began to lose muscular control and balance. His mother, Dot, who had seen films on television of BSE cattle stumbling about in fields and farmyards, began to get anxious that her son might be suffering from a similar disease.

At Newcastle University there was a young student called Peter Hall, who loved pop music and would make video recordings of himself singing to famous pop tunes. He fostered this image by keeping his hair very long in 1960s fashion. He took care of his hair meticulously, washing it virtually every day. Then his mother, Frances, noticed that his hair was growing lank. Her son had suddenly lost interest not only in his hair but also in pop music and even his studies. When the doctors were called in, they diagnosed depression.

Frances, an intelligent and concerned mother, had been aware of BSE and Sporadic CJD for some years and, despite government reassurances, had stopped feeding her family beef. These concerns resurfaced as she watched her talented and lively son fall into both physical and mental stupor. Anxiously, she asked her doctors if this could possibly be a case of CJD linked to BSE. Not a chance, they said. Put the idea out of your head – Peter is far too young to get CJD

There were other cases, too, in London, Glasgow and Edinburgh. In most of them, the medical response was similar. Whether or not this was due to simple medical caution I cannot prove but, being a doctor myself and having practised in my earlier days, I am only too aware of the pressures on a doctor when faced with an unusual and difficult case.

The chances of it being a highly unusual condition are slim, and to make such a diagnosis is to invite raised eyebrows amongst senior colleagues with the potential for ridicule should that diagnosis be proved wrong later. The normal procedure is to eliminate any other possible illnesses – of which there are many. This is a long and arduous process, after which one is forced to grasp the nettle and put forward a risky hypothesis. Because there was – and still is – no legal requirement to report CJD cases, and the diagnosis is generally proven only by a postmortem examination, it is not known how many people dying of paralysis and dementia are certified as having diseases other than CJD when this could have been the cause of death.

In 1995, there could not have been a doctor in the land, whether a country GP or a leading hospital consultant, who was unaware of the existence of CJD. They would also have been aware, from Vicky Rimmer's case, of the existence of a new form of CJD. Nor could any of them have been under any illusion about the hysteria that would be generated if they put forward such a diagnosis.

Whether or not they were reluctant to make a diagnosis is a matter for debate but it appears also that not all such infections were reported to the CJD Surveillance Unit in Edinburgh, as all doctors had been requested to do since 1990. Until her son's death, Dot Churchill had not even been told that there was such a thing as the CJD Surveillance Unit; when she discovered its existence herself, she contacted it personally. Some doctors may have been reluctant to report their suspicions; others may well have simply misdiagnosed a case, which would not be particularly surprising as it was such a new condition. I suspect, for instance, that over the years hundreds if not thousands of cases of Sporadic CJD in elderly victims have been diagnosed as the much more prevalent Alzheimer's Disease.

However, as the summer of 1995 turned into autumn, the Edinburgh scientists received reports of the half a dozen or so cases of the new disease in young people. This was in fact a spongiform brain disease, but brain scans of samples taken from the victims were showing a pattern of damage significantly different from that of traditional Sporadic CJD. In these scans, there was a much denser concentration of damage with areas known as 'plaques' surrounded by 'haloes' of PrP, the protein manufactured by prions. This arrangement of plaques and PrP haloes was much more similar in pattern to that of brain tissues of BSE cattle than that found in humans with the sporadic form of the disease.

These, without doubt, were the findings that the Edinburgh scientists had hoped they would never make. They had indisputable evidence of a disease never before recorded in human beings. And, given the similarity between the brain patterns in infected cattle and those of these new human victims, it was virtually impossible to deny that the two were connected.

Whether or not they did deny it I do not know – that, I hope, will emerge from the BSE inquiry. There was certainly no indication of any government response acknowledging these facts.

In October 1995, the front pages were full again of news that a fourth farmer, this time in North Wales, was suffering from what appeared to be a human form of BSE. A government spokesman said that this could not be confirmed until the poor farmer had died.

The furore that this statement rekindled in the media was so great that the biggest gun in the land was wheeled out to fire a broadside against the speculation which, once again, was having a devastating effect on beef sales. The Prime Minister, John Major, felt obliged to stand up in the House of Commons to announce: 'There is no scientific evidence that BSE can be transmitted to human beings'.

This was completely untrue. Up in Edinburgh, the CJD Surveillance Unit now had half a dozen cases which suggested strongly, even if it had not yet been proved conclusively, just the opposite. But driven either by scientific caution or by pressure from Whitehall, the Unit had decided that they could not publish such information until they had more confirmed cases of the new disease.

It was a statement that Major would live to rue for the rest of his time in Downing Street. I do not know the Prime Minister's motives in making it. I presume it was a last-ditch attempt to save the British beef industry and to placate our increasingly nervous and irritated partners in the European Union. He had always seemed to be an honest and decent man. It seems to me unlikely that such a man would deliberately lie in the House of Commons to fellow MPs and, via the television cameras, to the nation as a whole. If he was not lying, he was unaware of the Edinburgh findings which means, in turn, that he had been ill-advised by either his political colleagues or their civil servant minions at the Department of Health and MAFF.

In political terms it was rather like the last heroic stand the British army made on the beaches of Dunkirk before being swept into the sea. It may have been proclaimed as a victory but it was, in fact, to be proved by subsequent events to be a shattering defeat.

Anne Richardson, the 40-year-old mother from Liverpool, died in January 1996. Her husband Ronnie – the man who had been falsely accused of abusing her when she began to suffer unexpected falls in the house – was left an angry and bitter man.

Peter Hall, the music-loving student from Newcastle University, died the following month. A photograph taken of him soon before he died brings back the awful images of victims of Nazi concentration camps, his long, proud hair cut back, his once fun-filled eyes dark and lifeless in deep sunken pits. He died without a murmur, without a word of complaint.

Brain samples from both were sent to the CJD Surveillance Unit. By March, the scientists there dared hold back no longer. On 18 March, they flew to London after requesting a top-secret meeting with the Spongiform Encephalopathies Advisory Committee (SEAC), the government's advisory committee on BSE and CJD. There they gave a presentation, which included photographic slides of brain sections taken from eight victims of new-variant CJD, showing graphically that they had died from a new brain disease which, almost certainly, was a form of human BSE.

For the scientists and politicians, it was a day of quiet desperation. As one of the scientists told the BBC2 documentary, *Mad Cows and Englishmen*, two years later, 'I knew that this the worst day in British history since the Falklands War or perhaps even 1939.'

On 19 March, several key members of the SEAC committee were in Paris at an international conference on spongiform brain diseases; others were at their universities or going about their daily business. That evening, the Secretary of State for Health, Stephen Dorrell, was attending the opera at Covent Garden. He was called out take a phone call. It was the Prime Minister who, at last, had taken a decision about BSE that should have been made eight years before: the BSE crisis was to be taken out of the hands of the Ministry of Agriculture and would in future be handled by the Department of Health. And Dorrell would have to make an announcement to the House of Commons that a 'likely link' had now been established between BSE and human new-variant CJD.

The switch of responsibilities was, presumably, meant as a reprimand to MAFF and designed as a reassurance to the general public that, at long last, serious efforts were being made to control the spread of BSE into the human population. If so, it failed abysmally, as the government was to discover to its cost.

The SEAC committee – some of them called back from the Paris conference under instructions to make their sudden departures as inconspicuous as possible – was ensconced in a basement room in Whitehall with orders to come up with a plausible statement for Dorrell to make to the House of Commons. In the meantime, SEAC chairman, Professor John Pattison (who had replaced Tyrrell in autumn 1995), was at a meeting at Number 10 Downing Street, facing across the desk John Major and a group of people he did not at first recognize: he was informed later that they were the entire cabinet.

The cabinet had been called together that day to discuss future electioneering tactics: there was, at this time, a general election looming and the Tories were already taking a pasting in the opinion polls. Instead, they spent two hours grilling Pattison. There can be little doubt that even the least astute politician in that room feared that this new event threatened their chances at the polls.

Neither meeting came up with any concrete conclusions about what Dorrell's statement to the House should contain. After the SEAC meeting, one scientist turned to another as they blinked in the Whitehall sunlight and said: 'What a fucking disaster.'

When it comes to the plain, unvarnished truth, such language could hardly be bettered. But for Stephen Dorrell, who admits that this was his most difficult day ever in the House of Commons, some varnish did seem necessary. When he rose in the glare of the television lights on March 20 he said that there was a 'likely connection' between BSE and CJD but the government thought it wise to take 'further' precautions – the latter in my view laughable in view of the inadequacy of the government's precautions so far.

Then, much to the dismay of watching SEAC scientists, he added a piece of information which devastated them: an announcement would be made within days to make clear if children or young people were particularly at risk from eating beef. This, as Dorrell later told the BBC, was designed to deflect questions he expected from MPs anxious to reassure mothers that their children were not greatly at risk. However, that one remark caused more panic in the nation's kitchens than any single statement in the whole sorry BSE saga. Dorrell's whole statement confirmed to the public what they had long suspected: that their government had been lying to them, persistently and consistently for years; this remark suggested that children might be in particular danger.

Members of the National Farmers' Union were alarmed, but their feelings were mild compared with those of the SEAC committee. For Dorrell had seemed to suggest that there was to hand evidence about the risks of beef to children, either for or against. In fact, there was none – not a single scrap of it. And when it came to a heated press conference, Dorrell had to admit as much. As a result, as Jon Snow said when he opened that night's Channel 4 News, 'The government cannot give assurances that it is safe for children to eat beef.'

As Professor Pattison was to admit later, 'It was like lighting the blue touch paper.'

After my long battle, my theories had been vindicated. My reaction, though, was not one of satisfaction but one of profound sadness, anxiety and suspicion. I was sad at the waste of so many years and the terrible effects of that; anxious that the now confirmed cases of new-variant CJD might prove to be only the tip of the iceberg; and suspicious that, even after an embarrassment of such huge proportions, the government might somehow strive to turn BSE to its advantage.

I had, as it happens, been one of the few people in Britain privy to Dorrell's announcement 24 hours before he rose in the House of Commons, thanks to an enterprising reporter on the *Daily Mirror*, Kevin Maguire. It had been Maguire who had broken the story about young Vicky Rimmer, the first victim of a new form of CJD. On 19 March, he had been tipped off about the likely contents of Dorrell's announcement the following day, and one of his first reactions was to telephone me.

I took him step by step through the entire history, and described in considerable detail the symptoms that human victims would be likely to suffer. Then the Mirror asked me to write an article on my views about the handling of the BSE crisis. Both appeared the following day. The *Mirror's* front page headline was: 'OFFICIAL: MAD COW CAN KILL YOU – GOVT TO ADMIT IT TODAY'. My piece was printed on page two under a headlined message to readers: 'YOU ARE RIGHT TO BE ANGRY'. In it, I outlined details of the government cover-up and recommended that the opposition should press for an independent enquiry.

That day, I was on my way to give a lecture to doctors and other health professionals in the town of Dumfries in Scotland. As I was in my car heading across the M62, my mobile phone rang, the first of some 60 calls from newspapers, radio and television. Before I reached Dumfries, much to my relief, the phone battery was flat. Although by then I had become used to barracking from certain audiences, that night my audience seemed shocked into silence by the news of the day and my expressed fears for the future spread of BSE into humans. It was an indication to me of the severity of the stage this unfortunate saga had reached.

It would be pleasing to be able to write that the government's admission of a link between BSE and CJD marked the end of the beginning – for the beginning of the end, to quote Winston Churchill, is not yet in sight. Worst of all was the fact that young people continued to die of CJD, like Matthew Parker, whose case is described at the beginning of this book. And after the Dorrell announcement, another shameful period of the story began.

Faced with a massive loss of trust by the British public, and with a general election looming, the Conservative government might have been well advised to try to regain the public trust by putting in hand measures to prevent the further spread of the disease and find a cure. Instead, as I had feared, with stunning cynicism, it tried to use BSE to its advantage in another way, by playing the anti-European card.

Not surprisingly, our partners in the European Union (EU), country after country, incensed that they had been given the official line that BSE could not infect people, announced total bans on British beef products: not just meat but items like bull sperm, gelatin used in processed food and bone meal used as a garden fertilizer. (Now, the Department of

Health has banned the export of human blood plasma because of the risk that blood from donors might be contaminated by CJD prions.)

The United States and other countries joined these embargoes, and at this point I became involved in an incident that illustrates the near hysteria that BSE had created throughout the world. When Oprah Winfrey, the top American television talk-show hostess, discovered that cattle in the United States were still being forced into cannibalism by being fed rendered remains of their own species, she vowed in April 1996 that she would never again eat a burger for fear of contracting BSE. This produced a lawsuit from Texas beef ranchers saying that the remark had seriously damaged their trade. I was flown to Dallas, and gave a long statement to Winfrey's lawyers. Huge pressure was applied by the beef lobby – they even managed to have the case tried in secret, which would be impossible in the United Kingdom and normally unthinkable in the United States. Finally, after seven weeks of legal argument, Winfrey was completely cleared by the jury and as a result the Texas laws that prevent public criticism of beef are in chaos.

In 1996, the United Kingdom was now isolated from the rest of the EU and there were many Conservative MPs who believed that, by stirring up anti-European opinion, they might stand a chance of winning the coming election. To my disgust, John Major joined this campaign and began making speeches designed to show that the bans on British beef were imposed not on health grounds, but for the benefit of foreign farmers. He even declared 'beef wars' by applying the British veto to scores of examples of European legislation (for example, the enabling of new member states to be considered for joining the EU), many of which we had previously fully approved, some of which we had actually proposed.

This, of course, made the British seem a nation of fools and knaves in European eyes. But it seems to me that someone in Conservative Central Office was betting that stirring up anti-European feeling would serve another purpose: it would deflect British public opinion away from the fact that, for eight years, the BSE scandal had been allowed to drift because private commercial interests were put before those of the public health.

The realization by the public that they had been lied to brought about a massive loss of confidence in the Conservatives after 18 years in power. And they showed their disapproval in the only way they knew. There were, of course, a hundred other reasons for Labour's landslide victory in May 1997, but I am sure the double-dealing over the BSE affair was one of the key factors.

However, I do not want to finish this account of the BSE debacle on a political note. Commercial considerations first unleashed this deadly disease on the nation, and a political cover-up allowed it to flourish, but the most important point is that new-variant CJD is a public health problem. I hope politicians and the scientists in their employ will now accept this and sail full-steam-ahead towards reaching a solution. There is still a long and hazardous voyage of discovery ahead.

If CJD does, as I have predicted, turn into a full-blown plague, it will make the AIDS epidemic seem like a common cold. Billions of dollars, pounds and francs have been spent on research into AIDS, which with sad exceptions like the victims of infected blood transfusions, is largely spread by activity always known to have associated risks. At long last, positive results are beginning to show. Various drugs and vaccines have been developed which, if they do not prevent HIV turning into full-blown AIDS, at least slow down the onset of the fatal symptoms. In some cases, they seem to arrest that onset almost indefinitely.

As far as I am aware, as a scientist who has spent the last decade studying every known scientific report on spongiform brains diseases in both animals and human beings, no research on a similar scale is being carried out anywhere in the world on BSE, a disease spread by the simple and innocuous act of eating a meal. As Britain has the sad distinction of being the country which disseminated this terrible disease, and then allowed it to spread unchecked, we surely have a duty to launch such a programme now and carry it through with total determination and all the necessary resources it demands.

As yet, we do not even have a test to show whether people are already carrying an infection that, between tomorrow and 30 years from now, might sentence them to a disease which robs them of movement, speech, sight and laughter, and leads to a terrifying death. The sentence on their families and friends is months of torment before death and years of grief and nightmare memories afterwards.

Nor must we forget the CJD caused by the growth hormone, which came from the pituitary glands of humans who had died either in accidents or from undiagnosed illness. It must be established whether they were already carrying prions which had not yet had time to launch their full-scale onslaught.

Much of the groundwork on prions has already been done. Surely the United Kingdom has the scientists and the facilities to isolate the prion and stop its deadly progress?

Research by Stephen Dealler and myself, and indeed by the government itself, suggests an infection rate of between five per cent and more than ten per cent in infected cattle herds. Although no human would ever have consumed the amount of prions that would have been contained in the infected feed that cattle were subjected to up until 1988 or 1990 (depending on which government date one believes), if prions act like other, better-known, infectious agents, just one in a human being might be enough to set off its lethal chain reaction. And for many years before 1987, hundreds of millions of meals were eaten in Britain, any one of which, theoretically at least, could have been infected. The government finally admitted in 1997 that BSE is being transmitted from mother to calf, so even now the risk of infection remains.

Predicting future numbers of CJD cases is pure guesswork. Members of SEAC and the CJD surveillance unit think there could be up to 10,000. And it could well be many more because, since apparently healthy cattle can transmit BSE down to their calves, we now face the devastating possibility that human mothers can also pass on the infection to their babies.

I wait, if not for answers, at least for signs that answers to all the questions there are still about BSE are being sought. I am sad to say that, as yet, I see little evidence that the quest is underway.

In harbouring these deep misgivings, I reflect that, in the past, my work has been ridiculed by some, only to achieve final vindication. But in the case of new-variant CJD, I sincerely hope that my fears will be proved wrong.

Part Three

Keeping Poison off Your Plate

16

FOOD IN THE SUPERMARKET

Over the years, I have been accused many times of being a vegetarian with a personal axe to grind, a fanatic with some secret agenda to bankrupt farmers and butchers. Neither is true: my family eat a fairly normal diet, including lamb and pork, game when we can get it, poultry, eggs, fish and cheese. As a family which, however, has lived for so many years knowing about various types of food poisoning, we do everything we possibly can to ensure that our food is not contaminated. This means shopping carefully, storing food properly, handling it with immaculate personal hygiene, and cooking it thoroughly.

There are, however, some items which are banned from the Lacey kitchen. These include British beef, a delicacy much missed by my wife and daughters but sadly off the menu until such a time as science has come up with a way of testing whether cattle are prion-free and can be certified as being so. With Fionna and I still in our fifties, we may be incubating CJD from the years before 1989 when we consumed British beef. To feed beef to our daughters Miranda, now 23, and Gemma, 14, would be unthinkable. To believe the claims of the NFU, SEAC and the government that beef from animals over 30 months old is dangerous but aged 29 months is safe is quite ludicrous.

I was once invited to a National Farmers' Union function in what I thought was a gesture of handing me an olive branch. In fact, when I arrived, I discovered that beef was on the menu. I suspected (and was afterwards proved right) that NFU press officers were hoping to issue a press release saying that I had eaten the forbidden meat. Such a statement would have been taken as my endorsement of beef. It would also have branded me a hypocrite, so I took the only action available to me: I walked out.

This is my personal view. There are millions of people who continue to eat British beef in full knowledge of its potential dangers, just as there are millions of people who choose to smoke, drink too much alcohol and, indeed, drive a motor car, all activities which involve risks that might be far higher than that of catching CJD. That is their choice in a democracy and I will not try to dissuade them: my earliest and most vehement protests in the BSE crisis were concerned with the fact that people were not being given the information on which to make this personal choice; that they were being told that the meat was perfectly safe when, in fact, what evidence there was pointed the other way.

In accepting the fact that many people wish to continue consuming beef, I would still like to emphasize most strongly that there are some beef products which are still much more likely to be contaminated than others (although we do not know which these are). Most recent legislation was rushed into effect without proper scientific input: the order to remove beef from the bone was to many experts ridiculous, because all the evidence suggest that prions are carried round the animal's body in its bloodstream and, therefore, could be present in any part of the anatomy.

Cooking beef will not, unfortunately, kill BSE prions but it will, in most circumstances, kill other food-poisoning agents (found not only in beef) which can cause a range of symptoms from mild discomfort via considerable pain to, in extreme cases, death. These are mainly the so-called 'killer bugs' described in detail in Part One: salmonella, listeria, E. coli, botulism and the less severe, but much more common, campylobacter, which is estimated to cause some 600,000 cases of food poisoning in Britain every year.

Although E. coli is often present in the cow's gut, the others are more likely to get onto or into meat products by poor handling in either the abattoir or the processing plant, in transit, or at the retail outlet. One of the major causes for this contamination, and what makes it even more difficult to fight, is the process of mincing, which (as I said earlier) has the effect of burying dangerous bacteria inside the dish, protecting it from the heat of cooking, which regularly fails to penetrate the centre of the dish. Mincing is an invidious process, anyway, designed to make normally unsaleable parts of a carcass fit (visually at least) for human consumption.

This is why, in the Lacey household, the following products are banned: sausages that might contain beef, burgers and meat pies. This includes pork and the newly concocted lamb sausages which, unless they carry the words 'pure pork' or 'pure lamb', are allowed by law under present legislation to contain up to 20 per cent beef. But even pure pork and lamb sausages have been minced, which adds greatly to the likelihood of contamination as well as containing some pretty unpleasant ingredients: meat from the nose and ears, skin, bone and gristle. Eat them if you will, but always ensure that they are properly cooked in an open frying pan or under a grill – never in a microwave oven. This usually means ensuring that the centre is no longer pink but a word of warning: since various 'red meat' health warnings, manufacturers have been producing a paler type of sausage which, even when undercooked, does not show pink. The only way to overcome this is by cooking them until the skin is almost black.

Although sausages can be made wholesome by proper cooking, there is one item of food which, in my opinion, should be banned by law: the deep-frozen 'jumbo' burger, or 'quarter pounder'. Just as mincing makes this burger more vulnerable to contamination, the deep-freezing process makes it almost impossible to cook properly, because of its size: it is harder to cook the centre without burning the outside. In tests at our Leeds laboratory, we were never able to raise the inner-core temperature of a jumbo-burger to the critical +70°C temperature (known to kill all food-poisoning agents except BSE) without severely burning the outer layer. If I were asked to declare any one item of processed food as 'public enemy number one', it would undoubtedly be the deep-frozen jumbo burger.

That said, we humans do after all need to eat and, contrary to many regularly expressed opinions, I believe that we should eat well: food is one of the great joys of life. To show how we maintain that pleasure with the least possible risk, I think we should now take a tour of my local supermarket. As these palaces of modern living tend to be designed on similar, very clear patterns worked out by consumer-psychologists, its layout will be very similar to most of those in the United Kingdom, which are now responsible for more than 80 per cent of the nation's food sales. We shall shop department by department:

Fruit and Vegetables

These are amongst the best foods that one can buy – cheap, wholesome and rich in vitamins and some minerals. They provide the body with much-needed roughage, and modern research suggests that a daily intake of five portions of either fruit or vegetables can markedly reduce the incidence of a number of cancers.

Potatoes, once denigrated for causing obesity, are in fact an invaluable source of energy from carbohydrates and, particularly in children, can provide an energy source as a substitute for sugar- and fat-rich snacks like sweets and crisps. In doing so, they are actually a valuable slimming food. There is no need to be over-particular in choosing only fruit and vegetables which are bright and shiny: you may get bargain prices for items which appear to be slightly past their best but, when peeled, are still of excellent quality.

In some cases, this shiny, 'fresh' appearance has been produced artificially: many oranges are sprayed with wax to produce this shine. If you use orange or lemon peel or zest in a recipe, wash them thoroughly first. All fruit which is to be eaten with the skin on – apples, pears, plums etc – should be wiped with a clean, damp cloth first. Many will have been sprayed with various pesticides and fungicides, and traces of these will otherwise be eaten. Although in minute quantities these are unlikely to bring about a sudden illness, these toxic sprays have been proved to build up over a long period of time in kidney and liver tissue.

Another modern trend that causes me concern on health grounds is the growing prevalence of ready-made salads. These are often doused with mayonnaise, which is an ideal growth medium for harmful bacteria, as was proved in the fatal listeriosis cases in Canada described earlier. Knives or machines used in the slicing process can readily cause cross-infection. I recommend that you buy your own whole vegetables and slice them yourself at home using a clean knife. If they are to be stored with mayonnaise, keep them in a covered container in a refrigerator with a temperature of, at most, +3°C.

The Bakery

Many supermarkets now have their own in-house bakeries and produce bread and cakes of very high quality. Good bread, particularly wholemeal (as opposed to 'malted brown loaf' which may be merely dyed) is an excellent component of a healthy diet, providing energy from carbohydrates, minerals, a fair amount of protein and some vitamins. Because bread and cakes are 'dry goods' with little internal moisture, they are not good breeding grounds for infectious bacteria, making them one of the safest of our foodstuffs. Bread, like potatoes, is not inherently fattening unless eaten with large quantities of butter, cheese or, in particular, jams or preserves. Wholemeal bread is also a major provider of roughage. Discard all bread, of course, if there is any sign of mould.

Dairy Products

Here we are entering one of the food-poisoning minefields. Foods like butter, margarine and hard cheeses like Cheddar are low in inner moisture and therefore not good breeding grounds for food-poisoning bacteria. Most people store them in their refrigerators, but this is not necessary unless your house is kept very warm or there is a summer heat wave. They will store quite adequately, if well covered, at room temperatures. What is more, their taste will be enhanced.

Once again, however, modern fads and fashions have intervened to create potential health hazards. So-called 'low-fat' products have more internal liquid and, combined with the food itself, can be an ideal breeding ground for bacteria. These products should always be stored in a cold refrigerator and eaten by the sell-by date.

Worst of all, from a health point of view, are the soft cheeses like Camembert and Brie. Although acids used in the cheese-making processes will kill most known bacteria, these cheeses are left to grow a crust and, in the dairy and food store, are subject to regular handling. Any cross-infection caused by poor handling will provide that bacteria with an ideal growth medium.

My experiments with listeria in soft cheeses proved conclusively that these cheeses were a major danger to certain highly vulnerable groups: pregnant women, young children, senior citizens, people already ill with some other disease or injury, and those taking certain drugs like steroids. No one in these categories should ever eat soft cheese!

Sadly, the dairy-product minefield does not end there. Yogurts have been proved to be the cause of several food-poisoning outbreaks, including one involving botulism, perhaps the most dangerous of all the known food-borne bacteria. It is now possible to buy small units for the home-production of yogurt under conditions which you yourself can control. By using your left-over milk with this equipment, you will also obtain cheaper yogurt, but it is essential that your hygiene is impeccable.

Soft Drinks

Few parents realize that fizzy drinks like colas and lemonades can act as an ideal incubator for certain yeasts that can be dangerous. A bottle left with the screw top loose, or worse still, a half-drunk can of fizzy drink left at room temperature can cause quite serious illness, particularly amongst toddlers – whose appetites for these drinks seems insatiable. I would recommend the purchase of smaller bottles or cans, which are more likely to be drunk in one session.

This, I admit, is more expensive than buying large bottles, and if the latter fit the family purse, they should be sealed tightly and kept in a cold fridge: airborne yeasts can find their way into the most unlikely places but cannot multiply at very low temperatures. The best advice on these drinks, however, is to wean your children off them in favour of cordials or squashes made by adding water. Most modern fizzy drinks contain very high concentrations of sugar, which rots children's teeth and can lead to obesity in later life. Squashes will also, of course, contain sugar but in much smaller quantities when diluted.

Bottled Water

Another modern fad is for 'designer water,' a taste common for many generations in mainland Europe, where tap water was often polluted until comparatively recent times (and still is in many parts of Germany, for instance, because household supplies come from the heavily polluted River Rhine). This fashion has now spread to our shores and to the United States and, sad to say, most of the reasons behind it are simply poppycock.

Carbonated water – where the fizz is introduced artificially – does have some benefits from a health point of view. The carbonation process adds acids to water which will, in fact, kill most known infectious bacteria. There are, however, naturally fizzy waters that are prone to containing harmful bacteria, and one, French Perrier, only a few years ago was also proved to be contaminated by benzine, causing millions of bottles to be withdrawn from sale across the world. (The manufacturers say this is now safe.)

Bottled still waters are, frankly, a joke when it comes to public health. If their producers are to be believed, they too are drawn from natural spring waters which, like anywhere in the countryside, might be subject to many forms of pollution from animal faeces, naturally occurring minerals and micro-organisms, and the artificial pesticides and fertilizers used in large quantities by farmers. Unlike tap water from the mains supply, there are no regulations governing the purity of bottled water and few regular checks to ensure that these bottled still waters are free from contamination. They are far more likely to cause illness than water from the tap. I recommend putting tap water into a bottle and keeping it in the fridge so that is always cool. It will taste much the same and be a great deal cheaper.

Crisps

Here is another food product that presents untold numbers of parents with a difficult choice, thanks to multi-million-pound advertising campaigns often broadcast during children's viewing hours. The simple answer would be to ban crisps altogether – they are nutritionally questionable, bad for teeth and can lead to obesity – but in a democracy, people should be allowed to make these choices for themselves. To make this choice, they should be given adequate advice on the crisp-packet labelling. They are not.

There are basically two basic types of crisp, one made from potatoes deep-fried in palm oil, the other using different oils. Most caring parents reading crisp-packet labelling and seeing the words palm oil would, I believe, think them fairly wholesome: vegetable oils, as opposed to animal fats, are now perceived to be healthy. The truth of the matter is that palm oil is very high in saturates, the fats which, as in butter and cheese, are known to be major causes of cardiovascular diseases that can bring about heart attacks and strokes.

The reason why crisp manufacturers prefer to use palm oil is that it is very stable: it does not break down quickly and therefore keeps the product crisper for longer. Other oils, high in more healthy polyunsaturated fats, break down more quickly and the crisps become soggy. So guess which the manufacturers and supermarket chains prefer when that vital consideration, shelf-life, is at stake?

Despite dietary concerns, however, potato crisps, because they are essentially dry goods, are not likely to be breeding grounds for food-poisoning bacteria when they leave the store still wrapped. The trouble is, crisps are consumed with the hands by children who may be involved in other activities like using the lavatory, fondling pets, or playing in pretty grubby surroundings, such as a sand pit. The opportunities for surface contamination from the child's own fingers are therefore high: on a similar front, one of the more disturbing findings of a recent microbiological examination of peanuts left on a public bar showed they were likely to be contaminated with several samples of human urine from men who had been to the lavatory and not washed their hands afterwards.

If, therefore, your child must have crisps, I would suggest you allow them to eat them in clean surroundings after having properly washed their hands – indeed this should be done before any food is eaten by hand – and discard any crisps not consumed in a relatively short time.

Biscuits

Like crisps, these are essentially dry products, which do not provide a good breeding ground for bacteria. They do, however, tend to be high in sugars and fats and are therefore not a recommended part of a healthy diet if eaten in large quantities. One or two, however, will not do a child much harm, because children burn a great deal of energy in comparison to their body weight. A quick infusion of sugar and fat in a biscuit can replace used energy. Like crisps, however, biscuits should be consumed in clean surroundings and not left lying around.

Bacon

Bacon is one of the few modern foods which is still preserved, partially at least, by the use of salts and, in particular, sodium nitrite. To some health faddists, salt has today become a dirty word, yet it is one of the key food preservatives in human history because it prevents bacteria from multiplying. All human beings need a certain salt intake – in desert and tropical countries, the loss of vital body salts through perspiration or stomach upsets is a major cause of death.

Athletes and sportsmen and women playing high-speed games like squash or tennis in hot weather need to replace these salts as quickly as possible. All human beings also need a certain amount of fat to remain in good health.

Bacon provides both salt and fat and is highly resistant to bacteria. Because it tends to be cooked in thinnish slices at very high temperatures, either in a frying pan or under the grill, any surface contamination caused by poor handling or storage tends to be quickly killed. Never, however, cook it in a microwave oven. Bacon, then, is a highly desirable food taken in reasonable quantities.

Sausages

As I said at the beginning of this chapter, the Lacey family rarely eat sausages because firstly, we do not know what they contain, and secondly, there is no really efficient way of proving that they have been thoroughly cooked. It is, I think, significant that one of the most virulent form of food poisoning, botulism, takes its name from the Latin word for sausage, *botulus*.

If, however, you cannot resist the odd banger, choose either pure pork or pure lamb sausages, because legislation guarantees (as if any such guarantee can ever be 100 per cent binding) that they contain no beef. Better still, try some of the newer sausages made from game such as venison or even wild boar: these semi-wild creatures are much less likely to suffer from the cross-contamination often found in intensive farming units and their meat is also lower in saturated fats. They taste extremely good, too, which after all is one of the most desirable qualities of any food.

Eggs

Yet another minefield and one which, it is reasonable to estimate, causes hundreds of thousands of isolated food-poisoning outbreaks every year. My research suggests that one in 7,000 eggs is contaminated with salmonella, which may seem a very low proportion. If, however, it is realized that Britons eat hundreds of millions of eggs every year, this contamination rate adds up to very large numbers indeed.

It is, of course, a matter of personal choice for a healthy, reasonably young man or woman to decide if he or she should take the risk of consuming one of these infected eggs lightly cooked: I understand only too well the pleasure of a runny boiled or poached egg eaten with buttered toast. If such a choice leads to salmonella poisoning, the attack is likely to be uncomfortable rather than dangerous in the stated conditions of relative youth and good health.

I cannot emphasize too strongly, however, the risks of lightly cooked eggs to pregnant women, the elderly, the very young and those already ill or taking medication like steroids, which weaken the body's natural defence mechanisms. Salmonella can and does cause miscarriages in pregnant women. It makes young children seriously ill. And it is sometimes fatal to the elderly or sick.

So if you are a member of this high risk group, please cook your eggs so that both white and yolk are solid; the addition of a little butter or margarine will take away the dryness. Scrambled egg, so long as there are no liquid contents remaining, is a pleasant and safe way to eat what is, after all, a major staple food full of the vitamins, proteins and minerals needed by the human body.

No one, however old or young, fit or fragile, should eat home-produced food made from raw eggs and not cooked. Mayonnaise, in particular, has a long and sinister association with severe and sometimes fatal food-poisoning outbreaks. This does not mean that mayonnaise is off the menu for ever: commercially produced mayonnaise has been pasteurised and will be perfectly sterile until you open the jar. From that moment, it should be stored, the lid carefully tightened, in a cold fridge and consumed by the date shown on the labelling. If not, you have in your kitchen an almost perfect incubator for poisonous bacteria.

If that were not enough, there is one final warning about eggs which, I thinks, displays the cynicism demonstrated by some sectors of the poultry industry. Early in 1989, a massive investigation by trading standards officers of England showed that thousands of eggs marked 'free range' on sale in shops and supermarkets had, in fact, been produced by battery hens. This was, of course, nothing less than a fraud perpetrated on consumers concerned at abuses of animal welfare, who, to demonstrate their concerns, were willing to pay considerably more for eggs that they believed had been produced by hens living in fairly natural surroundings.

Unpleasant though this is, I am sorry to say that when it comes to the public health, free-range eggs, even if genuine, are more likely to be infected by salmonella than those from battery farms. The reason for this is that, in a battery farm, the egg rolls away from the mother as soon as it is laid and is taken away by conveyor belt. In free-range conditions, the egg may lie in infected matter for some time – as long as a week or even more – where it is likely to suffer slight cracks from the claws of the mother and other hens. Surface salmonella can penetrate the egg through these tiny cracks and begins its deadly replication.

These concerns have now been raised in the EU and new legislation is to be introduced in 2009 which will give battery hens – and other factory-farming victims like pigs – more humane conditions coupled with much tighter hygiene controls.

Until then, the only advice I can give for healthy egg consumption is: cook them until they are hard.

Sauces and Pickles

Here we have another of mankind's traditional preservatives at work: vinegar. Its strong acidity kills most known bacteria and prevents others taking hold in items like pickles, sauces and ketchups. Some of the sauces also have a high sugar content, which is also a natural preservative. However, once again, fashion and the profit motive have been stripping us of the protection of these ancient safeguards.

Many manufacturers are diluting the concentration of vinegars because a 'light' taste is now preferred. Sugar, which sucks moisture from a food by a process known as osmosis, makes that food less likely to support bacteria. But sugar and fat contents are being reduced to attract the slimmers' market. This means that many sauces that, a few years ago, could have been left for weeks in a kitchen cupboard without fear of contamination should now be stored in the fridge and used as quickly as possible after opening. The problem for the consumer is: which ones?

Food labelling, or rather the lack of it, is still to my mind a national scandal. What information there is tends to be minimal, scientifically confusing to the average consumer, and sometimes downright misleading. When it comes to a simple matter like a bottle of sauce or a jar of pickles, even I would find it difficult to judge how long they could be kept safely.

Pickles should, in most cases, be safe for cupboard storage because the vinegar concentrations are still relatively high. In sauces and ketchups, the information available is so misleading that the only safe method of storage is tightly sealed in a cold fridge. I would also recommend buying smaller bottles and jars, so that they are consumed more quickly, a piece of advice which I give with the greatest reluctance because it will add even more to supermarket profits: the smaller the item, the higher the profit margin. In these circumstances, the food manufacturers and retailers benefit by not labelling their foodstuffs clearly and concisely. Only the consumer loses.

Fresh Meat

This could be the biggest, widest, and most dangerous minefield of all. However, in addition to the observations made about beef at the beginning of this chapter, I will say that it is a minefield that can be crossed in perfect safety should certain simple rules be observed.

To prevent the better-known infections, meat should be cooked well by traditional methods – roasting for long periods, casseroling, or cooking thin slices under a very hot grill or in a frying pan at high temperatures. This will kill harmful bacteria causing surface contamination. Personally, I would never cook any meat or poultry in a microwave oven.

For those with animal welfare as well as health concerns, lamb is perhaps the best of the traditional meats. All sheep are raised in genuine free-range conditions, and are therefore less likely to suffer from cross-contamination. Lamb is still, however, vulnerable to surface contamination, so traditional cooking methods apply. If you are using minced lamb for, say, a shepherd's pie, simmer it gently for an hour or more and then, for the last few minutes, raise to a fierce boil and stir vigorously: this will ensure that all harmful bacteria are killed.

Pork, although produced by intensive farming methods, is not a natural carrier of many infectious agents dangerous to man, so long as it is cooked fresh and stored in a cold fridge before cooking. It can become dangerous if left in warm kitchens for longer periods. One warning, though: pork is a regular stir-fry ingredient. If you must use this method, make sure that the meat is cut into very fine pieces and cook it fiercely at very high temperatures for at least five minutes. The meat should be white, not pink, when eaten.

My family have taken up with relish some of the game meats that are now coming onto the market. Venison and wild boar have few risks if cooked by traditional methods. So, too, have game like pheasant, partridge, and hare. With beef off our menu, they make a safe and extremely tasty alternative. Being wild, they also tend to have a much lower fat content than battery-produced meats.

Poultry

Another major hazard if not cooked properly. Salmonella is, as I have documented, endemic in thousands of British chicken flocks, but it is also found in turkeys and, to a lesser extent, ducks. However, salmonella is easily destroyed by traditional cooking methods, although in stir-frying extreme care must be taken that the meat is cooked through completely, as with pork. There is one recent development which I would suggest everyone ignores: the arrival of the turkey burger. Here, once again, manufacturers are mincing a meat that can carry salmonella, greatly increasing the risk of protecting bacteria from cooking heat.

Even more dangerous, however, is the old British habit of stuffing poultry before roasting. Although I am usually in favour of traditional cooking methods, this one appals me for concrete scientific reasons. The fact is that any chicken, and many other poultry, will almost certainly be carrying salmonella within its carcass. To ensure that this is killed, it is essential that hot air in the oven penetrates the body cavity. Stuffing affords a dense layer of protection to the bacteria and is one of the most dangerous culinary habits on this island. If you want stuffing with your poultry, please, please cook it in a separate dish.

Frozen Foods

Another potential nightmare if not treated properly. In the supermarket, avoid packages which are 'sweating' on the upper layers of the freezer cabinet: they have no doubt been heated by the display lighting and, unfortunately, it is impossible to tell how long they have been kept in an unrefrigerated storeroom before being put on display. As most forms of bacteria easily survive the deep-freezing process, they might have already started the replication process when put on display.

Most consumers realize that the majority of frozen meat products should be properly defrosted before cooking. This means leaving in a fridge for at least 24 hours and, in the case of whole poultry, anything up to three days. Defrosting in microwave ovens is a hit and miss process, for it is almost impossible to discover if the centre of the meat is properly defrosted without cutting it open, a messy process which can considerably detract from the appearance of the food.

I would personally never eat so-called 'complete' frozen dishes that contain minced meat – items such as lasagnes or cottage pies – because here is an example of virtually every risk associated with any food mixed together in one package: mincing, deep-freezing and, in all too many households, cooking in a microwave oven. This highly undesirable mix of food hazards is further exacerbated by the fact that, in trials conducted in our Leeds laboratories, most instructions on microwave packaging woefully underestimate the times required for thorough cooking: the suggested 20 minutes more often than not turned out to be 30 minutes, with similar underestimates up and down the scale.

However, I recognize the fact that frozen convenience foods are often a boon in households with children where both parents are working, which is now the norm for millions of families. Sadly, I can offer them little comfort except to suggest a cooking routine for this type of food: first defrost the dish for at least as long as the instructions suggest; then cook it in the microwave on high for another ten minutes; then put it in a hot traditional oven for another ten to twenty minutes.

This is laborious and often makes the food taste foul. In fact, it often would be quicker for the cook of the household to make an alternative dish by traditional methods, like grilling or, a highly recommendable process, in a modern steamer. The food would be safer, tastier and a great deal cheaper.

All this said, there are a few items of frozen foods which are of extremely high quality. Peas, for instance, are frozen literally within hours of being picked and not only taste very well but still contain useful nutrients and vitamins which leach away with long storage. However, in the huge range of products on the market, the recommending of a few peas barely represents a whole-hearted endorsement of the frozen-food industry.

Cook-chill Foods

If I can raise little enthusiasm for frozen food, the latest creation of the food-processing industry leaves me on the verge of despair. Admittedly, the campaign of my Leeds University team against listeria did bring about major improvements in cook-chill technology. But it is still open to so many types of infection from so many different sources that I find myself unable to recommend it in any way.

For healthy young people, needing to pick up a meal on the way home after a hard day at the office, it is perhaps a necessary evil. For the vulnerable groups I have already mentioned, it is something that should be avoided: they would be better to open a tin, which would be cheaper and a great deal safer. Canned food has been heated to temperatures which will kill all viruses and bacteria. Unless left opened for some days before being consumed, canned food is one of the least likely causes of infection we know.

Fish

Finally, one of my favourites. This is not only an extremely important part of any balanced diet, it is also one of the safest: in natural conditions, fish carry few bacteria which can be harmful to man. People in places as far apart as Japan and the Mediterranean, to whom fish is a major source of protein, also consistently suffer from lower incidences of so-called Western illnesses like cardiovascular problems and cancers.

As well as being packed with protein and highly beneficial oils, fish is usually cooked at temperatures high enough to kill any surface contamination. It also comes in so many shapes, sizes and varieties that it is a gourmet's delights. Although many high-street fishmongers have been put out of business by the big supermarket chains, many of those supermarkets now provide excellent fish counters.

Even here, however, there is a need for some caution. Fish farming, mainly of salmon and trout, has now become big business. These fish are generally fed on cereal and poultry pellets, which could themselves be contaminated with harmful bacteria, and are also routinely dosed with chemical products (as described in chapter ten). These I tend to avoid for two reasons: partly due to the possibility of chemical contamination, partly on moral grounds, for I find it offensive that creatures like the magnificent, ocean-going salmon should spend their lives cooped-up and crowded in cages – which are also now becoming an increasingly worrying source of marine pollution.

There are problems, too, with shellfish if not absolutely fresh. A close friend of mine once poisoned his entire family – wife, children and himself – by serving *moules marinières* with mussels bought from his local fishmonger. He and his wife were in bed for a day with intense stomach pains and his children were ill for three days. Mussels often feed in waters heavily polluted by human sewage outlets into the sea.

Although it is illegal to harvest such a crop in most of these areas, one can never be sure that those laws have not been broken.

Additionally, all fresh shellfish should be alive when bought. If they have died during harvesting, during transit, or on the fishmonger's slab, they can begin to decompose rapidly and become a source of toxins. Anyone preparing shellfish should immediately discard any with opened shells.

Lobsters, crabs and prawns tend to have been cooked in boiling water within hours of being caught, the process which gives them their distinctive pink colour. So long as they have not been kept on display for too long, they should be totally wholesome. Ask the fishmonger when the delivery was made: a shopkeeper keen to protect future business will usually give you a straight answer.

However, few of us dine regularly on lobster or crab. For a working mother, a budding executive on the way home from a hard day at the office, even a university professor back from the laboratory, there is an excellent and nutritious meal available on thousands of street corners in Britain: the creation which started the fast-food habit, fish and chips.

As I wrote earlier, eaten with a freshly prepared salad – mushy peas, I'm afraid, have little nutritional value – fish and chips cooked in vegetable oil are both nutritionally sound and bacteriologically safe. In all my career, I have never investigated a case of food poisoning connected with this most British of fast foods.

17

FOOD IN THE KITCHEN

Spotless as your kitchen might seem, it is here unfortunately that you are most likely to cross-contaminate food which, on arrival home from the supermarket, may be 100 per cent wholesome. Poisonous bacteria are, of course, completely invisible to the human eye – in fact, they can only be seen under the most powerful of microscopes. Millions could live and multiply on a spot of grease or other nutrients the size of a pin head. But there is no need to live in a constant state of anxiety about kitchen hygiene if certain basic rules are understood and adhered to.

Personal Hygiene

The first thing to understand is that one of the most likely sources of contamination is you, the cook. With today's busy lifestyles, the ordinary human being can pick up harmful bacteria from almost anywhere in the environment: on the train or on the bus, in the garden or by stroking a pet, at the office or in the house itself. It goes without saying that after using the lavatory, everyone should thoroughly wash their hands. But having done so thoroughly, it might still be possible to pick up another infection from the next doorknob you turn.

Hand Towels and Dishcloths

The first thing to do on entering the kitchen is to wash your hands again and dry them on a clean towel kept aside for that sole purpose: to wipe your hands on a tea towel used for drying crockery or cooking utensils is asking for trouble; to wipe them with a wet dishcloth is positively dangerous, for dirty dishcloths are a notorious source of cross-contamination.

Dishcloths should be washed thoroughly, and preferably scalded, after each washing up session and discarded after a few days. Perhaps the easiest way to avoid dishcloth contamination is the use of cheap disposable ones on sale in any supermarket. Paper towels will perform the same function for drying hands after washing: the clean sheet torn from a kitchen roll will be totally sterile – unless it has been kept in a place where it can be contaminated by food remains – and will only be used once.

This is, of course, more expensive than using traditional cloth towels and dishcloths but these too can be kept perfectly safe if they are properly laundered and changed regularly.

Kitchen Surfaces

Many consumers concerned at hygiene risks have begun to buy antiseptic solutions to be sprayed or wiped onto kitchen surfaces. These are, in fact, an expensive waste of money as long as all working surfaces are cleaned regularly after every meal with hot soap-and-water and, preferably, a scrubbing brush. It is essential, of course, that all spots and stains from food are carefully removed and the brush should be allowed to dry out thoroughly before being used again: without moisture, any bacteria it has picked up will die.

However, even in the best-cleaned kitchens, there are danger areas: areas of tiling that are cracked or where the grouting has fallen away; ill-fitting joints in surfaces; nasty nooks and crannies in corners or under cupboards. These should be resealed using specifically made sealants, available from any DIY shop. Check them regularly to ensure that no new cracks have appeared and, if so, reseal them immediately. These cracks and crannies make ideal food traps where bacteria can breed at leisure.

Knives and Utensils

If not properly used, these can become the ideal means for transferring bacteria from one food item to another. One of the most dangerous actions that any cook can perform is to trim the fat from a piece of raw meat and then use the same knife to chop a lettuce for a salad. Raw meat is perhaps the most likely single item of food to suffer from surface contamination, and should always be treated as a potential source of infection.

In the cooking process, that surface contamination on the meat will be killed. But it may have been transmitted from the knife to the lettuce. If that lettuce has been kept in the open and is moist, it can become a breeding ground. If it has been covered with mayonnaise or some other rich dressing, the cook has created a veritable incubator for high-speed replication of infectious agents.

I would recommend the professional chef's practice of having a series of knives for different foods: meat, vegetables, fruit etc. But even then, the knives should be rinsed regularly under very hot water and dried on a clean cloth (preferably paper kitchen towel) between different chopping and slicing actions.

Raw and cooked meats combine to create one of the major threats to kitchen hygiene. Raw meat, as I have emphasized, should always be treated as though it carries surface contamination. If blood or scraps from raw meat come into contact with cooked meats like ham or tongue, the potential for very serious cross-contamination becomes truly alarming. This was almost certainly the cause of the *E. coli* outbreak in Scotland (detailed in chapter seven) that killed more than 20 people.

So the previous advice about knives becomes doubly important here. Either use a different knife for carving raw and cooked meats or, if the same knife must be used, ensure that it is washed and dried with the greatest of care. Raw and cooked meat should also be stored carefully, as described in the section on refrigeration below.

Chopping Boards

These, too, are a dangerous source of cross-infection. Personally, I would recommend the use of two different boards: one for raw meat, and one for all other ingredients. Mark them clearly, or buy two different types, so that you know which is which. I realize that this is not a cheap option, for even one good chopping board is an expensive item. For cooks whose pockets are not deep enough for such luxuries, the chopping board should be washed with liquid soap and very hot water and scrubbed well between each operation – tiresome but, I believe, absolutely essential.

There is also one more vital decision to be taken here: any chopping board that has become badly scored should be immediately discarded. Those old knife marks can be an ideal breeding ground for bacteria. However, using antiseptics on a chopping board is quite unnecessary if the previous advice is followed. These are not as effective as proper hand cleaning.

Pets

Food should never be left uncovered on kitchen surfaces where it can attract the attention of pets. Cats will get almost anywhere, of course, but there are many breeds of larger dogs which can stand on their hind legs to steal food left uncovered. If these animals have recently been out in the garden, their paws may carry many different forms of bacteria, quite apart from the fact that these animals can also carry diseases harmful to humans. Cat litter trays should never, ever, be sited in the kitchen.

Pests

Flies, cockroaches and other beetles can and will invade any kitchen where there are scraps of waste food to be found. They can, of course, be killed by pesticide sprays and powders, but I have a built-in distrust of using strong poisons in the proximity of human food. The best advice here is to keep flies out by means of secure window frames and, if needs be, fly screens (you can, of course, always swat them with a newspaper).

Storage Cupboards

Many foods normally stored in the refrigerator can be kept happily at room temperatures so long as your kitchen is not inordinately warm: ideally, room temperature should be kept as low as is comfortable, for it will become warm as soon as cooking begins. Foods that can be kept at room temperature include eggs, traditional butter and margarine and hard cheeses. 'Low-fat' butter and margarine substitutes should however be kept in the fridge. There are several processed foods that can also be stored at room temperature safely even when opened, such as pickles with a heavy vinegar concentration.

Most dry goods, such as flour, biscuits, rice and pastas, can also be kept safely in cupboards with one proviso: once their original packaging has been broken, transfer them to plastic containers with tightly sealed lids. The reason for this is not so much bacteriological contamination – dry goods like these do not offer the liquids which most micro-organisms need to replicate – but invasion by various mites and other tiny creatures which, if allowed to spread, can destroy large quantities of food. Badly packed food can also attract the unwelcome attention of mice and cockroaches.

Most foods will taste better kept this way and, in the case of eggs, be easier to cook. But always cover such foods to keep out dust, air-borne yeasts, flies and, of course, those ever-hungry pets.

The Refrigerator

The absolutely essential precaution here is to store raw meats, including poultry, on the bottom shelf of the fridge. If they should leak blood, which often happens despite modern supermarket packaging, this can cause highly dangerous cross-contamination with other foods. Any blood which leaks onto the bottom of the fridge should be very carefully cleaned using very hot soapy water and, again, the trusty scrubbing brush.

Cooked meats should be kept to themselves on a higher shelf. Fish should be very carefully wrapped when kept in the fridge – to contain the smell as much as anything else – but should not be kept for more than two days at the most for it deteriorates very quickly in taste and quality.

As for salads, fruit and vegetables, it seems to me a nonsense to keep these items in the fridge: as a keen gardener, I spend much of my time protecting my vegetables from frost; to put them into a frosty environment for storage seems a strange contradiction. These should best be kept in a cool pantry, the garden shed or even the garage. A cellar, if you are lucky enough to have one, is ideal. Should you like your salads crispy and cold, pop them into the fridge half an hour before serving.

All these measures, when it comes to using the refrigerator, are so far matters of common sense and simple practice. There are, however, grey areas that demand more careful thought. And they, few readers will be surprised to hear, largely arise from modern industrial food-processing measures.

There are many products that are perfectly safe until they are opened. These include mayonnaise, sauces and ketchups, jams and other preserves. Many people still keep these in the cupboard after opening, and this may be satisfactory in most cases. Some, however, carry a warning on the label saying 'Keep refrigerated after opening' and this advice should be strictly adhered to.

Many other processed food products, however, do not carry this warning, but I feel that they should be stored in the fridge anyway. Apart from being cool, the fridge if regularly cleaned and defrosted according to the manufacturer's instructions, also provides important safeguards: it will not be invaded by pests, it keeps out dust, and even if air-borne yeasts float in when the door is open, they will not replicate because the temperature is (or should be) too low.

So my final piece of advice about the household refrigerator is: buy a fridge thermometer. Ideally, your fridge should be kept at a temperature no higher than +3°C. This will not kill harmful bacteria – nor will your deep-freeze – but it will ensure that they will not replicate at high speed.

The Freezer

You can buy freezer thermometers and my recommended temperature would be between -18°C and -23°C. If there are ice-crystals on your food, this is a good rule-of-thumb indicator that it is cold enough (although you may never find these in a 'frost-free' freezer, however cold it is). A deep-freeze will not kill harmful bacteria either; like the fridge it will only ensure that they will not replicate at high speed – but foods at this temperature will never 'go off' – the bodies of mammoths frozen in Arctic ice 10,000 years ago have been discovered, and their meat was still edible when thawed. Deep-frozen food will, however, begin to lose flavour and texture after only a few months, so I do not recommend prolonged storage.

If you freeze your own food, like home-cooked meals or garden produce, please ensure that they are securely wrapped in heavy-duty film or, better still, put in plastic containers: frozen food becomes brittle and, when badly packed, small pieces can break off and fall onto other food. This could become a source of cross-contamination when the food is defrosted.

Defrosting is, of course, one of the critically important operations in frozen-food cooking. I would never eat any dish made in such a way that, on defrosting, I could not reach the very centre to ensure there is still no frozen portion remaining. This, in all my career, has been the most common source of food poisoning. If you buy ready prepared meals with instructions saying 'Best cooked from frozen' do just that: but add at least 50 per cent to the recommended cooking time using conventional cooking methods. I would never, ever, eat any deep-frozen food which has been cooked solely in a microwave oven.

And, for all the reasons I have explained elsewhere, in chapters four and seven, under no circumstances ever deep-freeze ready-prepared cook-chill foods bought from supermarkets.

The Kitchen Stove

Here I admit to being a traditionalist: an Aga or similar range that offers long cooking periods for often-cheaper cuts of meat is one of my ideals. But any traditional stove, whether gas or electric, is unlikely to be the source of infection, as long as elementary cleaning procedures are undertaken: carefully wipe away any deposits of fat or burned food – preferably whilst still warm as this will make the job easier. Cleaning the oven, I admit, is one of the nightmare tasks of most cooks but the reassuring message here is that ovens become so hot that they will kill virtually all known food-poisoning agents with the one sad exception of the BSE prion.

The Microwave Oven

This, I admit, is my *bête noire*, perhaps the single biggest cause of the great upsurge in food-poisoning cases in the past two decades. In our Leeds laboratories, we were rarely able to raise the inner-core heat of prepared microwave dishes above the critical +70°C for two minutes, the absolute minimum to ensure that bacteria was killed.

As I have repeated *ad nauseum*, I would never eat a ready-prepared frozen or cook-chill meal reheated in a microwave. This does not mean, however, that there is not one of these appliances in the Lacey kitchen.

However, it is used for a very small and selective number of tasks. It will, for instance, prepare quite good scrambled eggs – so long as the eggs are cooked until they are solid. It is also a quick and efficient way of preparing bedtime drinks using fresh pasteurised milk.

Most of all, our microwave is used for the reheating, within a matter of an hour or so (i.e. not long enough for bacteria to multiply), of food that has already been thoroughly cooked by traditional methods. If you have family members who come and go at different times, or have the occasional dinner party guest who arrives late, this is a useful adjunct to a busy kitchen. Let it become master of your culinary needs, however, and you have a monster in your kitchen.

Gadgets

There are now so many of these available that to describe them all would demand a book in its own right. I will, however, mention just two. One I treat with some suspicion, one is something of a boon in a busy household.

The former is the now-complex food processor, which can mix and liquidize many foods in a few grinding minutes without the benefit of bacteria-killing heat. This is, to me, potentially dangerous, because any raw ingredients could be contaminated and the action of the processor, like that of mincing, would do nothing more than spread and bury the infectious micro-organisms throughout the food.

My second reservation is that the various blades and other moving parts in these processors are extremely difficult to clean properly: to do so thoroughly by hand adds longer to the overall time involved than if the cook had chopped the ingredients by hand using a properly cleaned knife. If you use these gadgets, ensure that the ingredients are properly cooked afterwards. To use them for raw dishes is taking a risk.

There is, however, one newish gadget which has my thorough approval: the dishwasher. There are some environmentalists who disparage their use because they do consume considerable energy and, in their early days at least, a great deal of water. Today, there are models on the market which are greatly more efficient in both electricity and water and, from a hygiene point of view, they do a very good job. Because of the pressure of the hot water used, and the high temperature of the hot air used in the drying process, they tend to get plates and dishes cleaner than washing by hand. Few bacteria could survive in such an environment.

There is, however, one word of warning: soak pans and dishes with heavily burnt-on food remains and scrape these away before putting them in the dishwasher. This way, your dishes, pans and cutlery will be about as clean as is possible outside laboratory conditions.

Waste Disposal

Left-over food remains are one of the most potent sources of bacteriological replication. Efficiently disposing of this waste is one of the major problems in restaurants and other mass-catering establishments – and also a regular source of food-poisoning outbreaks.

In the domestic kitchen, these problems can be overcome by a few simple steps. Always make sure your kitchen waste bin has a tightly sealed lid to keep away flies, other insects, and, of courser, those nosy pets. Always have a plastic bin-bag inside the container. Never fill the container too full, and always seal the bin-bag before putting it in the dustbin, which should be done at least daily and more often if there is a lot of waste. The waste bin and the dustbin should be regularly disinfected.

Finally, after dealing with any kitchen waste, always wash your hands.

Good food is one of the great joys of life, one of the joys which the Lacey family enjoy on a daily basis. In preparing it and cooking it, we tend to favour the older ways, the methods that our ancestors developed by trial and error over thousands of years. You can, however, use some of the modern ways in safety if you follow these simple rules. *Bon appetit!*

18

FOOD IN THE FUTURE

In the first three months of 1998, when, as my three-year contract with the small Leeds hospital ran out, my career as a NHS microbiologist was reaching its end, and as I contemplated my future, other food concerns were beginning to arise. The potential impact of biotechnology and genetic engineering began to sink into the public mind; at the same time, reputable organizations with concerns about the public health were bringing anxieties about new farming practices back into public debate. Ironically, these were issues that had been causing me considerable worry – which I had been expressing – for some years. Pleased though I was that these issues were being aired, I hoped that in facing them we would not repeat the mistakes of the food scares of the past.

Early in the year, the National Consumers' Council (NCC), a government-sponsored body under the wing of MAFF, issued a long report about the dangers to human health caused by intensive farming and the ever-increasing use of growth hormones and other drugs on livestock and poultry. The NCC was also worried about the increase in the use on farmland of nitrate fertilizers, which were leaching into the human water supply. At the same time, the Royal Society for the Prevention of Cruelty to Animals was giving a cautious welcome to EU proposals for the introduction of improved conditions for battery hens and farm animals right across Europe – cautious because these proposals, even if accepted, will not come into effect until the year 2009.

All this was taking place whilst talks were underway which will allow mainly agricultural countries in eastern Europe, such as Poland, to join the now 15-strong EU. Even in its present state, the EU can produce much more food than we can possibly consume, a situation which has led to the growth of absurd policies such as 'set-aside', under which thousands of farmers are paid millions of pounds *not* to grow crops on parts of their land. This had created the ludicrous situation that, on the areas of land which they were allowed to cultivate or graze, even more drugs and fertilizers were being used to boost production.

Other threats to the safety of our food were coming from what, next to computer research, has been the biggest growth sector in American big business in the last ten to fifteen years: biotechnology and its scientific bedmate, genetic engineering.

In the past, all great advances in agriculture and horticulture have usually come from two sources: either new breeding or husbandry techniques developed by practical, hands-on farmers and breeders, or agricultural scientists working in universities or government research bodies. Britain has played a proud part in both areas: it was the 'Improvers' of the eighteenth century and later who developed, by careful cross-breeding, many of the breeds of farm animals and varieties of crops which, until recently, were the bedrock of our farming. British agricultural scientists played a major part in the 'Green Revolution' that has allowed mankind to continue feeding the majority of the world's burgeoning population. Both sources, pragmatic and scientific, had in common the fact that the results of their work were made freely available to other farmers anywhere in the world. New techniques, new breeds or new crops could be used freely for the general benefit of mankind.

In the 1980s, this mutual self-help largely ceased. As Reaganism flourished on one side of the Atlantic and Thatcherism on the other, publicly funded research was drastically cut in the drive for what was called greater government efficiency. Few areas of research can be more important than the effect on our health of the food we eat, but on both sides of the Atlantic, public funds for it began to dry up. The neuropathogenis research unit in Edinburgh, for instance, had been faced with closure until the BSE scandal erupted and saved it, and it became associated with the CJD research unit. Into that vacuum, mostly in the United States, marched big business.

Billions of dollars were poured into this new field by private investors. This may seem insignificant: if the research is done, it may be argued, is it not better that it comes from businessmen than from the public purse? The answer to that is, sadly, no, for there is one crucial difference between the benign developments in food production in the past and this new era of research based in Silicon Valley and elsewhere: now, these scientists are doing it for profit.

In this sinister situation, certain new foodstuffs or animals are being *patented*. In other words, any farmer who produces them or any consumer who eats them has to pay a royalty to the company which produced them. Those who cannot afford to pay will therefore be denied the food. In the West, food consumers will see their food bills rise. In areas of Africa and Asia where starvation is rife, whether these foodstuffs, which could perhaps save thousands of lives in the short term, will be distributed will depend on the whim – and the profit margins – of those investing in them.

Let us consider the first products of this privately financed food research to come on to the market: irradiated food and genetically engineered food.

Irradiated food has been the subject of one 'scare' which is, in fact, unfounded. The practice of irradiating food by bombarding it with gamma rays gave rise to speculation that such food would be radioactive and therefore toxic to consumers. This, in fact, is quite untrue: the gamma rays leave behind no source for future radioactivity.

But, at the same time, its long-term costs to the consumer have been largely ignored. What the gamma rays do is kill bacteria within fruit, vegetables, chickens and prawns – the items already subjected to this treatment – which first bring them to ripeness, in the case of fruit, and then begin the decomposition process. The financial motive for this is shelf-life. Food that passes its sell-by date has to be destroyed (or, in many cases, sold on to other outlets like market traders). This is a costly business, and any measures to cut such costs are welcome in the cut-throat world of the food supermarkets.

By halting the decomposition process, irradiation keeps an article like a strawberry looking succulently red and shiny for up to two weeks rather than a little over two days. When applied to many types of food, such a time difference can add millions to a supermarket's bottom line. But it can bring dangers, too: recently, a cargo of prawns brought to Europe from the Far East was found to be heavily contaminated with cholera bacteria. Though the prawns had been irradiated, which killed the bacteria, later tests showed that the toxins manufactured by the bacteria were still present.

Moreover, what neither the irradiation scientists nor the supermarkets' own highly trained food experts tell the public is that fruit and vegetables reach their maximum flavour and food value at the very moment when ripeness has peaked and the fruit or vegetable is beginning to decompose. This is the time when the food not only tastes best but also contains the highest concentrations of natural sugars, vitamins and other nutrients beneficial to the consumer's health.

Irradiation seeks to postpone this peak of flavour and wholesomeness. Anyone tempted to buy an irradiated strawberry because it looks so delicious is being misled. Millennia of experience have taught human beings to judge the best time for harvesting and eating fruit and vegetables. By presenting irradiated fruit and vegetables that have not reached that optimum time, yet look ripe enough to eat, the modern food industry is undermining that judgement. What is more, the consumer has to pay more for a strawberry that has not reached its best possible flavour in order to cover the costs of expensive irradiation treatment.

Irradiation, then, is a trick which can also pose risks to the public health. Its dangers, however, pale in comparison to those potentially presented by the genetic engineering of food and, in particular, of food animals.

The process of genetic engineering is so complex that it could only be fully explained in a book devoted entirely to the subject. Its overall aims, however, can be simply stated as being the changing of the characteristics of a plant or an animal by removing a gene or genes from its DNA and replacing them with genes from another plant or animal. In this way, the human race now has the power to create new life forms which would otherwise either have taken millions of years to develop by natural selection or, in the majority of cases, would never have evolved at all. For example, it will soon be within the power of man to genetically engineer a cow with flesh that tastes like chicken or even fish. Such cows could grow to the size of an elephant and therefore produce large quantities of this new-tasting meat – a prospect that might seem highly profitable to farmers, or rather agri-businessmen as many farmers might now be more accurately described, in the third millennium.

Throughout this book, I have referred to organisms that can live in symbiosis with one host yet cause dangerous, and sometimes fatal, illness when transferred to another. In most cases, the victim is the human being. This is a fact that had been known to scientists, doctors and veterinarians for decades. Now, just as we threw away the wisdom of ages in the ways we cook and store our food, we are in danger of discarding this knowledge in the pursuit of profit. To tamper with the genes of any living organism is to tamper with the future. The scientists in the brave new world of biotechnology are, by creating new life forms, playing God; but they have not yet proved that these life forms cannot become host to some as-yet unknown form of disease. The fact that we now know to our cost that an organism which was utterly unknown to science only 30 years ago, the prion, is capable of jumping from species to species and changing its own physical characteristics each time it crosses the species barrier (with the result that BSE in cattle causes new-variant CJD in humans) shows that it is impossible to foresee what dangers lie in store. Bacteria, viruses and organisms like the prion have shown that they are capable of keeping pace with developments brought about by man. Regularly, as with the prion and the HIV virus that causes AIDS, they have shown that they can actually outpace our ingenuity and take advantage of a new set of circumstances well before we are able to develop countermeasures, causing immeasurable suffering in many parts of the world. If we continue to create new life forms artificially, we lay ourselves open to the possibility of similar unimaginable dangers.

These concerns are not the lone ramblings of a so-called Mad Professor. These concerns are shared by thousands of scientists around the world, and by millions of ordinary people. Even politicians are getting worried.

When scientists in an agricultural research centre near Edinburgh announced they had produced Dolly, the first ever cloned sheep, one very important person took notice: Bill Clinton, President of the United States. Said to be a consummate politician when it comes to feeling the public pulse, Clinton set up a commission to study the whole problem of genetic engineering and threats, if any, it presented to the future. Since then, some of the finest brains in the world have been pondering the scientific and moral uncertainties created by genetic engineering. Many of these uncertainties share a common theme, asking where should we draw the line, what research is acceptable and what should be banned.

In assessing genetic engineering in relation to public health issues, it seems to me that there are three main criteria to examine: firstly, is the research potentially dangerous; secondly, can its objectives be reached by other means, and thirdly, will the general public benefit in the long term?

My fears on the first issue I have already expressed. These fears suggest that, in the case of the second issue, if a desirable objective can be reached by using techniques other than genetic engineering, the former should be given preference. The third is more complex.

There are certain areas of genetic engineering where the means can be said to justify the ends. For instance, researchers have been able to engineer a bacteria that can naturally produce large quantities of insulin for human use in cases of diabetes. This insulin is identical to that produced naturally in the human body, unlike the pig and cattle insulin that has been used until now. Such advances could be of untold benefit. So, too, could experiments which allow animal organs to be used as donor organs for heart, kidney and lung transplants in sick or injured human beings; donor organs from humans are always in short supply. But these advances cannot be made before science has solved the problem of these donor organs taking with them new viral infections to the human recipient.

However, the pouring of millions of dollars into research to produce, for example, a cow that tastes like chicken would be, to me, a scandalous waste of precious scientific resources. It is inherently dangerous, as I have explained, yet, in pandering to tastes rather than enhancing health, it achieves no justifiable public benefit.

Before my career petered to an end, there came one final savage twist in the BSE scandal. I was following with great interest the reports of the BSE inquiry set up by the new government under the chairmanship of Lord Justice Phillips, a distinguished High Court judge. On the very first day he had asked for permission to extend his reporting time to 18 months: there was too much work to be undertaken, he said, to complete the report sooner, and he had no wish to come to any decisions or recommendations without the most thorough of investigations. This, I thought, was a sign that the inquiry would be no whitewash.

As the reports of the early proceedings came out day by day, I could not help indulging myself with some wry smiles of amusement as the politicians, scientists and vets who, for ten years, had seemed united in defending the handling of the BSE problem against my criticisms began to blame each other for the disaster that followed. Even Sir Richard

Southwood, author of the infamous and now discredited 'dead-end host' theory, was forced to admit that he had been pressured by MAFF not to recommend any actions 'which would increase public expenditure'. This was the first public confession that the interests of the public purse had been put before that of the public health.

I was invited to give evidence and submitted a 37-point detailed account of my attempts to bring the scandal into the open. However, I received my summons to give evidence with some misgivings, for I saw that I was due to appear on Tuesday 17 March, budget day. Budget day is, by tradition, the day when any government chooses to issue bad news unconnected with financial affairs. The reason is that the newspapers the following day, and the broadcast media on the day itself, are so brimming over with budget news that other matters largely escape attention. Cynically I decided that the choice of the date of my summons had been made deliberately to ensure that little of my evidence would be reported. I became apprehensive that, despite the new government's declaration of more public accountability, my old foes at MAFF were still pulling the levers of power to silence me.

Then, on the Friday before my appearance, came a strange incident. It began with a call to my laboratory from a man with a strong Geordie accent who asked if he could come to see me at my home on a matter 'that I would find of the greatest interest', which he was unwilling to elaborate further on the telephone.

I was, of course, curious, but I was also more than a little concerned. I had been subject to death threats over previous years and that weekend I had addressed a meeting of farmers in north Wales that became so threatening that I had to be taken away under police escort. However, as always, my curiosity got the better of my personal fears, and I invited the man to my home. He duly arrived, accompanied by two other men, and the subject they had come to discuss was, indeed, a matter of great interest.

My caller was what was once called a knackerman, a man who visits farms to take away dead cattle and other animals and makes his living by selling what parts of the carcass still have value: the skin for leather and the bones for glue and bonemeal. One of the other men was also a knacker; the third was a renderer who made his living from rendering down cattle carcasses. Once, all three men had made a good living by

204

offering their services to farmers. Now, BSE regulations had made cattle carcasses virtually worthless and they had been forced to start charging the farmers for their services, instead of performing free or even paying for dead carcasses. As a result, business had begun to dry up.

This, of course, was not an unfamiliar tale to me: thousands of rural businesses have run into bankruptcy as a result of the government's mishandling of the BSE crisis. However, their story had a new twist: they told me that to dispose of dead cattle, some farmers had taken to burying dead carcasses in shallow graves in remote areas of the Highlands, south-west Scotland and the north of England. Proving this, they had photographs – hundreds of them – and, most significant of all, video tapes.

Many of the cattle had been buried near streams and burns flowing into major rivers, which provide part of the human water supply. I knew from statistics that one of the areas shown in the many photographs, the Grampians region of north-east Scotland, had the highest incidence of E. coli poisoning per head of population in the United Kingdom. The possible link between dead cattle, the water supply and E. coli gave cause for urgent concern.

I assumed that the farmers were burying their dead cattle merely to avoid paying the knackers for taking them away. But at this point in the conversation, one of the trio corrected me. Many of the buried cattle, he said, had died from BSE. That very week, the EU had lifted the beef ban on cattle from Northern Ireland in herds which had been BSE-free for eight years. Anticipating that the ban on beef from Scotland would in due course also be lifted, with the same stipulation, some Scottish farmers, said my informant, were prepared to give up the compensation payments for destroyed BSE-infected cattle – which have been progressively reduced and may now be as little as £200 per animal – rather than report that they had a BSE case in their herd, and they were therefore burying cattle that had died from BSE. They also receive something like £650 for a suspected BSE animal which, after tests, is proved to be free of the disease, encouraging unscrupulous farmers to send off a healthy animal for compensation and secretly bury the diseased ones.

I thanked my visitors and after they left I thought through the implications of this information. The video and photographs showed hundreds of dead cattle with parts of their bodies protruding out of their shallow graves. If some of these cattle were indeed BSE victims, the whole BSE extermination policy in large areas of Scotland was under threat. If this were happening on such a large scale in northern Britain, it could well be happening in southern England and Wales. Furthermore, predators and carrion eaters would be having a field day: foxes, stoats, wild mink and rats, plus several species of carrion-eating birds, would doubtlessly be gorging on these beef carcasses clearly showing above ground. It was also highly likely that domestic dogs and cats from outlying farms would be joining the feast. Cats and mink, we already know, are hosts for the prion; it is possible other species could be. Should other species become infected in the wild, this deadly chain might spread even further.

Packing up this evidence in my briefcase, I left home to board the train which would take me to London and the BSE inquiry.

Budget day 1998 was a day of two parts: one in which I was proved right, the second in which I was proved wrong.

Despite my fears that as I was called to give evidence on Budget day attempts were being made to suppress anything I would have to say, as soon as I arrived at the entrance to the BSE inquiry building I began to sense that this might not be so. A jostling pack of press and television journalists and cameraman besieged me and, for the first time in many years, they seemed to be genuinely interested in comments I might like to make, rather than subjecting me to a barrage of loaded questions designed to make me appear as the Mad Professor. My written evidence, already submitted, had been issued to the press, and so they believed they knew, more or less, what I was about to say. They were in for a surprise.

I began to reveal my new evidence about the illegal mass graves in Scotland. I explained that the significance of this was that not only was there a risk of BSE infecting other species in the wild but, even more sinisterly, it also raised grave doubts about the accuracy of government figures, according to which the rate of the incidence of new BSE infections was falling rapidly – now down to some 2,000 a year, well below the 1993 peak of 36,755.

Within hours, these facts were on the front pages of evening newspapers and leading radio and television news bulletins throughout the country. The suggestion that farmers were deliberately fiddling the BSE figures by carrying out these mass burials soon reached the ears of the NFU officials. Without asking to see any of the photographs or the video, they denied the existence of the graves. One official said that it was 'absurd' to suggest that farmers would deliberately hide BSE cases because, in doing so, they would deprive themselves of compensation payments. The following evening, Channel 4 News led its evening broadcast with film of the shallow graves, showing clearly the exposed remains of dead cattle. I had been proved right, but it was a victory that gave me little pleasure.

My pleasure, indeed a feeling bordering on euphoria, came in being proved wrong. For at the BSE inquiry, Lord Justice Phillips and his colleagues, instead of trying to destroy my evidence, as I had expected, allowed me four hours to explain the long, sad story of how, in my scientific opinion, the BSE saga had moved from cock-up through to cover-up.

I realized that Phillips and his two colleagues had read many of the scientific papers I had studied in the previous ten years, as well as the long study of the problem published by Stephen Dealler and myself in the *Journal of Food Microbiology* in 1990. This was, at the time, the longest and most detailed analysis of the potential threat of BSE to humans ever published. I told the inquiry that Stephen and I had personally paid for an extra 5,000 copies to be printed which we circulated to MPs, scientists and leading figures in agriculture and the food processing industry. What had been the result of these efforts, Lord Justice Phillips enquired? Nothing, I replied. The paper had been completely ignored. The judge and his colleagues made a note of this answer.

By this stage of the proceedings, I was becoming aware that I was getting, for the first time, a fair hearing from people who had studied the facts with great care. They even had a full transcript of my appearance before the House of Commons at which, bullied, badgered and angry, I had stated that, in the worst-case scenario, new variant CJD might wipe out an entire generation of people in the twenty-first century.

Lord Justice Phillips began to read from the transcript.

'On what evidence did you give that reply?' he asked.

This was the question I had not been asked by the Select Committee. I had been longing ever since to put the answer on the public record.

'There was an outbreak of TSE on a mink ranch in America in 1965 in which every single animal died,' I replied. 'Those mink had been fed on cattle waste. When I gave my reply in the House of Commons, I had that case in mind.'

Lord Justice Phillips sorted through the pile of papers on the table before him. 'Ah yes,' he said. 'We have a report on that incident here.'

I can only describe my joy at that reply as sheer elation. Anyone who had read the report on the 100 per cent fatality rate in that American mink outbreak would have understood my House of Commons reply, given when I had been asked to predict the worst-case scenario. But the Select Committee had either not read that report or chosen to ignore it.

At last, I had been given the chance to put the record straight. At last someone was listening – a man who seemed anxious to collect all the known facts without political fear or favour. I almost danced my way out of that chamber.

But whatever the outcome of the inquiry, sadly, I have no doubt that the previous government's mishandling of the BSE crisis means that the number of new-variant CJD cases will continue to grow in the next 20 years or more, and that many families will have to undergo the terrible suffering of seeing their loved ones fall victim to this dreadful disease. Research findings now emerging show that new-variant CJD affects only people with certain genetic similarities, so a large section of the population will, it is hoped, be spared. Tragically, however, an estimated 18 million are still at risk if they have been or are to become infected.

If such suffering is to be avoided in future, we must launch the most extensive research programme ever carried out in this country, to isolate the BSE prion and find a means of defeating it. We must discover a method of testing people who may already be incubating new-variant CJD in the early stages. We must find ways of comforting and curing people in the latter stages of the disease.

Although it may be of little comfort to the victims, it is nonetheless important to say that the whole BSE scandal must become a warning to anyone with responsibilities towards the food we eat that public health must always have priority over politics and profit. There are many lessons to be drawn from the scandal by many different factions. Some of those lessons are already being learned.

As I write, there is a rash of supermarket-chain mergers underway or under discussion in the City of London. The reason for this is that over a period of almost 40 years, the relentless expansion of supermarkets has been at the expense of small, independent food retailers on our high streets, not only putting thousands of small businesses into bankruptcy but also blighting the centres of our cities, towns and villages. This process has now reached the point of self-destruction: with the opposition virtually wiped out, the supermarket chains can now only fight amongst themselves. Furthermore, environmental pressures against car use will increasingly make out-of-town shopping more expensive and less acceptable socially. Faced with decreasing profits, the major food retailers might at one time have been tempted to introduce more highly processed foods, which are cheaper to produce, but, with the constant threat of food scandals, they will now be less likely to do so. A welcome consequence, I predict, will be the decline of the supermarket within 20 years or so, and the return of the small high-street butcher, baker and greengrocer.

For major food processors, BSE and all the other food-poisoning scandals must act as a salutary warning. No longer will they be able to get away with using meat without knowing whether or not it is safe, or be able to take any risks in the preparation of food. The public are catching on to potential dangers in food and are demanding higher standards. To ensure its future survival, the food business must put quality and hygiene before profit.

For farmers, I have much sympathy – they, after all, brought about the spread of BSE in total innocence: neither they nor scientists know where BSE first originated. Until BSE is eradicated the British beef industry must, I am afraid, look forward to a long period of decline. Faced with this dismal prospect, I believe farmers should begin to look for other products and crops, and here there is a huge opportunity. With an ever-expanding EU, to which many of the newer entrants are largely rural, Europe's problem will be one of producing too much food. This coincides with growing public awareness of the need for a healthy diet and the dangers, both moral and medical, of intensive farming, in which live animals are kept in conditions akin to concentration camps, and our fields and rivers are polluted with fertilizers often toxic to wildlife.

The opportunity for farmers, therefore, is to produce less food of higher quality. Let the poultry and the pigs grow up and breed in open fields; look for new livestock that produce healthier, lower-fat meats, such as venison, boar and even ostrich; let us grow more fruit and vegetables under organic conditions – not only do they taste better but they will make our countryside a healthier place for its wild inhabitants. If British farmers could make these fundamental changes, their way of life would, I believe, be profitable and they would also earn the gratitude of their town-dwelling customers. To farmers (although it may surprise them to hear me say so) I give my best wishes for the future.

I wish I could say the same about politicians. On them I reserve judgement, but there are many encouraging signs for the future. The establishment of the Food Standards Agency is a major breakthrough. The BSE report, when it appears, may expose once and for all the dangers of political interference in the science of food production and distribution. If this lesson is well and truly learned, no politician will ever again put the nation's health at risk for political gain.

Finally, the consumer. We all must eat every day, and eating should be one of life's major pleasures. We have a right to eat food that will enhance, not endanger, our health. Our best weapon in ensuring we get this is knowledge. We must keep ourselves informed and, armed with that information, use our power as consumers to ensure that the food available to us is good food.

In this book I have, I hope, done what little I can to point out the pitfalls that can put poison on our plates. Now, as I go into enforced early retirement – but honoured with the title of Emeritus Professor by Leeds University, a title I will carry for the rest of my life – I do not know what my future will be. I hope it will not be necessary for me to speak out again about food poisoning. Meanwhile I have a large and wild garden to tend, my orchids and my cacti to nurture ....

Appendices

These appendices consist of material already used elsewhere in committee, in court, and in another publication. As such, they appear as they originally appeared: spellings, phrasings, or stresses have not been changed to match the style of the rest of this book. Every effort has also been made to preserve the appearance of the originals in layout.

APPENDIX ONE

THE BSE INQUIRY

Statement of Professor Richard Lacey
3 March 1998

1. The purpose of my statement is to describe, from the time when BSE was first identified, my actions and statements about BSE and nv CJD and the reasons for those actions and statements. I have a number of criticisms about what was done about BSE and CJD. In this statement I shall describe the criticisms which I made at the time. I have other criticisms, which I have submitted to the Inquiry and I understand that they will be investigated. In this statement I describe only what I said and did as a matter of historical fact.

2. In order to understand the context it is necessary for me briefly to describe my role in food contaminations, other than BSE.

3. I qualified as a Doctor of Medicine from the University of Cambridge in 1964 and a Doctor of Philosophy from Bristol University in 1971. I then specialized in both child health and microbiology in London, Bristol and East Anglia. I have been Professor of Clinical Microbiology at the University of Leeds since 1983 and a consultant to the World Health Organisation since 1984. I attach as Annex 1 my CV together with two lists of my publications. It is my career function to prevent infectious disease and I have had a particular interest in preventing diseases in people that are derived from animals and food. In that capacity I advised the Ministry of Agriculture on the Veterinary Products Committee on matters concerning the use of drugs in animals, birds and fish between 1986 and the end of 1989.

4. One of my career roles has been responsibility for diagnostic microbiology laboratories that receive samples from ill patients. The rising incidence of salmonella and other food poisoning, listeriosis, prompted me and my Department in Leeds in the mid 1980s to research the reasons why this was occurring, with a view to trying to reverse the trends. It was evident from the outset that there would be a conflict between the interests of the food producers and that of the consumers, particularly as both these were the responsibility of the same Ministry. I have adopted the attitude that fear of such a conflict should not be a deterrent to researching, analysing and raising the issues. The outcome of this research has in some areas been gratifying with hazards from listeriosis, cook-chill and microwave use, now considerably reduced compared with 10 years ago. Unfortunately food poisoning from salmonella has remained high. The concerns, which I expressed from 1988 about salmonella in eggs inevitably led to criticism from the egg farmers and their Parliamentary supporters. Similarly when I made known my concerns in 1989 about processed foods, including cooked chicken, soft cheeses and cook-chill food, this led to similar people disparaging me. I also pointed out at this time that *E. coli 0157* was a potential problem with cooked meat. Therefore I was aware that with this background, raising the profile of BSE would generate anger from those with a vested interest. Despite that, my training and professional responsibility required me to give priority to the welfare of the public.

5. I did not take any significant interest in the emerging reports on BSE until I was researching for my Penguin book *Safe Shopping, Safe Cooking, Safe Eating* in early 1989. As part of my research for my book I read the official statements from the Ministry of Agriculture, and what I said in my book about BSE was the official wisdom of the Government of the day. I refer in particular to pages 162 to 164 of my book (Annex 2). The process of publishing the book in June 1989 however made me re-evaluate what I had written. I read the source material on which the official line was based and I now describe my thinking as it developed during the latter part of 1989. It was at this time that my family abandoned British beef as part of our diet.

6. The first document which I consulted was the *Veterinary Record* article published in October 1987 (Wells *et al*). The crucial information was that this was a new disease likely to be infectious in the major source of the country's food.

7. I next turned to the report of the Southwood Committee (February 1989). I came to the view that the report was essentially flawed in that the bulk of the report described BSE as a transmissible spongiform encephalopathy, that is a disease due to an infectious agent with the inevitability of the potential to spread to further members of the same species, or indeed to other mammalian species. Yet the report's conclusions considered that cattle were a 'dead-end host' for the infection, that is that it was non-infectious.

8. I also consulted the article by Drs Holt and Phillips in the *British Medical Journal* (1988). My reaction at the time was to share their concern about a new infection of the sort to which people were known to be vulnerable.

9. In August 1989 I expressed the view that the chance of BSE going to any member of the human population at all was around 5%, in an interview with James Erlichman, the Consumer Affairs writer of the *Guardian*, who was writing a general article in *Country Living* about food contamination.

10. The report of another Government Committee, the Tyrell Committee, was published in January 1990. The Committee recommended that the number of people succumbing to CJD be monitored over the next 20 years. At the time I thought that monitoring of a disease incidence was much less important than taking action to avoid the risk. Even at this time there was no cessation of infected herds breeding, there was no quarantine and there was no adequate documentation of most herds.

11. I became dramatically involved with the BSE issue when I took a chance telephone call from a London radio station on 10 May 1990. I was asked if I would give a telephone interview with a Mr Andrew

Neil who was rehearsing as a part-time radio presenter. I agreed, little realizing that the Andrew Neil in question was Andrew Neil, the then editor of the *Sunday Times*. We talked about food matters in general, including BSE. I explained that the numbers of cattle confirmed as having BSE were still rising, implying that BSE must be spreading between cattle and that all the infected herds should be destroyed. On the next day, a journalist from the *Sunday Times* telephoned and I repeated these comments. On Sunday 13 May the paper carried the front-page headline 'Leading food scientist calls for slaughter of 6m cows'. The next day, 14 May, the telephone at work never stopped ringing.

12. The consequence is that during the course of the next few days, the Government issued several News Releases and in addition the Minister for Agriculture, Mr John Gummer, made a statement to the House of Commons on 17 May.

13. The Agriculture Committee then decided to hold an inquiry into BSE. Mr Jerry Wiggin MP, the Chairman of the Committee, requested that I prepare a report on BSE and related issues for its Inquiry. I did this in collaboration with Dr Dealler who was then working in my Department in Leeds. Our memorandum is appended to the Committee's report. We entitled it 'The risk to man'. As I later explained to the Committee, we had only four actual clear days to produce a 30-page document.

14. I was asked to give evidence to the Committee on 13 June, along with Professor Mills, Dr Helen Grant and Dr Gareth Roberts. I did not know, until the morning of the hearing, who my colleagues at the hearing were. The transcript of the proceedings is in the Committee's report. Although I was not happy with the tone of the questions put to me by the Committee, nor with the fact that they spent time pointing out that in our rushed memorandum I had one extra word, nevertheless I was satisfied that I had put across the points which I wished to make and that there was a sound foundation to them. In particular my comment 'if our worst fears are realized, we could virtually lose a generation of people' (at page 55

of the Committee's report) was based on the well-documented instances of almost 100% of all mink succumbing to spongiform encephalopathy following eating contaminated feed. My fear was that it could happen to us if British beef carried the BSE agent and human beings were vulnerable to it. It was also evident at this time that most people had consumed contaminated beef and it was not then known that only a proportion of the population was susceptible to TSEs.

15. On 10 July 1990, the Agriculture Committee deliberated and the chairman, Mr Wiggin, read out the draft report. The report included a passage about my evidence, which suggested that I had seemed to lose touch completely with the real world when I said that we could lose a whole generation of people. I have indicated above the reasons for my comment.

16. Dr Dealler and I have collaborated on a series of articles on BSE and in addition I have been the sole author of some. The first of these articles was entitled 'Transmissible spongiform encephalopathies: The threat of BSE to man' which appeared in *Food Microbiology* in December 1990. We concluded that there was a distinct possibility that man could acquire spongiform encephalopathy from consumption of contaminated beef.

17. I repeated my concerns over contaminated beef in a book published in 1991 called *Unfit for Human Consumption*. At Annex 3 are pages 90 to 116 of this book. Table 10 is important as I summarized the particular features of BSE as I saw it in 1991.

'Features of BSE
Scale of epidemic unique to British Isles. Cows affected with clinical disease more often than cattle.
Most prevalent in S.W. and S. England.
Not known whether vertical transmission occurs to calves.
Not known whether humans are vulnerable.
The distribution of infectious agent is not known.
Rendering plants/protein supplements responsible.

Source of infectious agent possibly cattle.

Beef could be infectious agent for humans.

Uncertainties over infectivity to humans may persist for many years.

Cats have probably acquired the disease from cattle products.

More positive action required; it may be forced by economic pressures.'

19. I wrote a letter to the *Veterinary Record* which was published on 15 February 1992. This is at page 136 of my *Mad Cow Disease* book (published in 1994). The letter concerned the incidence of BSE. I relied on information given by the Ministry of Agriculture and which was published in *Hansard*. My conclusion was that BSE was now an established endemic, even though it was initiated or aggravated by feeding offal to cattle. I wrote my letter because of the revelation that the ages of the confirmed cases had dropped. The editor of the *Veterinary Record* provided a copy of my letter to the Ministry before publication to allow an instant response, also on 15 February. The response is at pages 137 to 138 of *Mad Cow Disease*. Mr Taylor, the Assistant Chief Veterinary Officer, pointed out correctly that the figures for 1989 were for England and Wales, and those for 1991 included Scotland. But in my view that was not the issue. It was the proportion of three year olds of the total that mattered. I did not of course include the 1,623 instances where the age was unknown. It was not my responsibility that the reporting and recording of ages was so sloppy that it yielded so many with 'ages unknown'. In my opinion it was scientifically correct to exclude data that has no meaning. It would not have been appropriate to add on the 1,623 cases to the total because it was not known how many were three year olds. But even if I had included these cases, the total became 19,620 and the percentage of three year olds becomes 15.3, still well up on 1989, rather than down. I considered that it was very significant that Mr Taylor did not dispute the accuracy of the yearly figures as presented, even though 'incomplete'. The remainder of Mr Taylor's letter defended the feed hypothesis and the line that due to accident or carelessness many cattle had probably received meat and bone meal when they should not have done. I was most 'impressed' as to how this information was obtained some years after the events.

20. On 13 February 1992 James Erlichman, the journalist, published an important article in the *Guardian*. The gist of the article was that the farmers might have used old feed for perhaps 8 weeks after the feed ban. In my view that was probably a red herring. The key observation was that one dam had given birth to 4 calves all of which subsequently went down with the disease, but the dam remained healthy, despite sharing the same feed. In my view, the most likely explanation is that the dam had been sub-clinically infected, with vertical transfer to each of the four calves, which later died of BSE.

21. David Hinchcliffe, the MP for Wakefield, asked a Parliamentary Question on 12 June 1992, on my behalf requesting details of the animal experiments carried out for the Government. I was surprised that Mr Soames, one of the junior Ministers of Agriculture, did not give any details and did not publish that information in *Hansard*, where it would have been available to all. Rather the information was placed in the Library of the House. Mr Hinchcliffe provided me with the Table which I now produce as Annex 4 as it appears in page 144 in my *Mad Cow Disease*. In my view the data was self-explanatory. Of most significance for the potential threat to man were the findings in the pigs and marmoset monkeys whose tissue proteins are similar to man. Also of relevance to potential human infection is the incubation period of the disease in the short-lived primate, the marmoset, with a high dose of brain directly inoculated, which was 4 years. This suggests that the incubation period in man, assuming vulnerability, would be seven-fold longer e.g. 12 to 50 ...

22. In early 1993 I asked Dr Tyrell for a meeting because I was dismayed about the lack of action taken to control BSE. On 22 June 1993 I attended a meeting with Dr Tyrell, Messrs. Bradley and Wilesmith of the Central Veterinary Laboratory and Dr Dealler (whom I asked to come with me). The meeting took place at the National Agriculture Centre, Stoneleigh. At Annex 5 is a record of this meeting which Mr Bradley prepared and which both Dr Dealler and I have agreed may be supplied to the BSE Inquiry and put into the public domain. I should point out however that despite initiating this meeting I had

not been informed of the existence of the minutes nor had I seen a copy until 26 February 1998. As I told Michael Elliot, the presenter of the documentary *Mad Cows and Englishmen*, there was no scientific dialogue. The Government scientists, Wilesmith, Bradley and Tyrell, were not prepared to consider the points that Dr Dealler and I made. I obtained the impression that the Government scientists were unable to consider our points as they were playing a predetermined role. I would particularly like to draw the Inquiry's attention to the danger of cattle bones (summary point 7 in the minutes of the meeting).

23. I published a contribution to the debate in the *British Food Journal* in July 1993 entitled 'BSE: The gathering crisis'. For some time, I had been puzzling why BSE cows typically succumbed at around age 4–5 whereas most cows were slaughtered at age 6–7 years. If infection was in their food throughout life, would the disease not be expected to occur most frequently following the greatest exposure; that is at age 5–6 years, not 4?

24. In September 1993 farmers began to contact me because they owned youngish cattle which they confidently believed were suffering from BSE. Farmers from all over the country told the same story. They had not kept possibly contaminated feed for months or years after the feed ban. On many occasions, the young BSE animal was born after July 1988 from a dam that had subsequently also succumbed to BSE, with the clear implication of vertical transfer. The Ministry vets thought otherwise. At this time I also gave several presentations to local authorities about the dangers from beef because the Meat and Livestock Commission had mounted a vigorous defence of British beef for school children.

25. In the autumn of 1993 I became concerned that the Government was massaging the figures for BSE cases by back-dating deaths to earlier years. *The Lancet* on 25 September 1993 said that 51,875 cattle died from BSE between 1988 and 1991 but on 26 November 1992 a House of Commons answer to a question from Mr Hinchcliffe said 48,526 died in that period. I alerted James Erlichman to the discrepancy

who published a story about it in the *Guardian* on 2 October 1993. He quoted me correctly as saying that presumably some recent cases of BSE had been added to the previous years to falsify the epidemic. I said that we needed an independent inquiry into the true state of the epidemic. According to Mr Erlichman, the Ministry accepted that there was a significant discrepancy, but the figures reported in *The Lancet* related to the date at which farmers first reported symptoms, while the deaths in the Commons answer were logged by the dates when veterinary surgeons ordered animals to be slaughtered.

26. The Ministry also suggested that the figures supplied to *The Lancet* included cases on the Channel Islands and the Isle of Man. I asked Mr Hinchcliffe to ask a question (*Hansard*, 1 November 1993) about the BSE cases for the Isle of Man and the Channel Islands. I set out the history of this in *Mad Cow Disease* at pages 151 to 153. The explanation of the Ministry did not add up.

27. Also in November 1993 Mr Hinchcliffe asked a further Parliamentary Question on my behalf. He asked the Minister for Agriculture how procedures for isolating, monitoring and reporting BSE livestock suspects born after 18 July 1988 differ from those born prior to that date. Mr Soames's answer, which I reproduced at pages 139 to 140 of *Mad Cow Disease* made me very concerned. In my view the effect of the change in procedure in February 1992 was to distort the number of BSE cases, with the inevitable reduction in the numbers of young animals slaughtered and confirmed.

28. In November 1993 Dr Stephen Dealler published a substantial appraisal of the total number of BSE cattle (including the numbers slaughtered before the onset of the terminal brain disease), the presence of tissue infectivity and the risk to the human population. He published this in the *British Food Journal* and it was entitled 'Bovine Spongiform Encephalopathy (BSE). The potential effect of the epidemic on the human population'. Among Dealler's estimates were that 7% of British cattle born in 1988 were infected with BSE, some 230,000 animals. Very many animal organs would have been infected, including many not within the group of banned specified

offals. In particular, liver, kidney and heart, which are commonly used in sausages and other, processed foods. I was proud to be responsible for editing Dr Dealler's article for the journal.

29. The *Veterinary Record* published a letter from Dr Dealler and myself on 5 February 1994 (which I reproduced at pages 166 to 168 of *Mad Cow Disease*) in which we cited an index case of a female Friesian-Holstein calf born on 4 July 1989, nearly a year after the ruminant feed ban. The events were precisely predictable from the changes in procedures to which I refer in paragraph 27 above. MAFF veterinary surgeons had told the farmer that the animal was suffering from 'ketosis' which is a non-specific chemical finding (too much acidity in the blood) in many illnesses. It usually tells you nothing other than that the animal is ill. The farmer then contacted me, as he did not accept this diagnosis. Subsequently the animal was slaughtered and the head was removed. The brain was processed at Grange Laboratories, Wetherby and examined at the Cambridge Veterinary School and at the Central Veterinary Laboratory. The diagnosis was 'typical BSE with severe spongiform change'. We wrote that the case history was strongly suggestive of vertical transmission of BSE. I add that the visiting veterinary surgeons would have been quite happy for the carcass to enter the food chain (with the exception of specified offals) and that this would have occurred had not the farmer contacted me.

30. Our letter in the *Veterinary Record* led to a published reply in the journal from Mr K. C. Taylor, the Assistant Chief Veterinary Officer in the Ministry, and to correspondence in February and March 1994 between Mr Bradley, the BSE Co-ordinator for the Ministry and myself. I set out this correspondence at pages 169 to 173 of *Mad Cow Disease*.

31. I had been concerned for some time about the thinking of MAFF that sheep scrapie was the cause of BSE. I asked myself why the Ministry had not tested their hypothesis experimentally in the UK. So I asked Mr Hinchcliffe to ask a Parliamentary Question in May 1994. Mr Soames answered on 17 May that no experiments involving the

inoculation or feeding of cattle with infective material from sheep with scrapie had been undertaken in Great Britain. Yet I learned from an announcement by the Ministry on 30 June 1994 that experiments, as late as January 1992, had in fact taken place, and that they had showed that the experimental feeding of calves with infected BSE material had resulted in the infectivity in the guts of those calves.

32. I continued to collaborate with Dr Dealler. During the course of 1994 I published with Dr Dealler an article entitled 'Bovine Spongiform Encephalopathy: The increasing threat to the human population' in *Rapid Methods and Automation in Microbiology and Immunology* edited by Spencer and Newson. We also published an article in *Human Reproduction* entitled 'Vertical transfer of prion disease'. We pointed out that prion diseases were vertically transferable in many mammals including man. We reanalysed the Kuru data which showed that the disease was prevalent mainly in adult women and in adolescents of both sexes and we proposed that this was due to vertical transfer and that this would explain why Kuru had not become extinct following the cessation of cannibalism, and raises the probability of vertical transfer of nv CJD in the human population.

33. In November 1994 my book *Mad Cow Disease: The history of BSE in Britain* was published. Following immediate hostile comments by Ministry veterinarians in *The Times*, no book shop stocked it.

34. In 1995 I published an article in the *Journal of Nutritional and Environmental Medicine* entitled 'Bovine Spongiform Encephalopathy – The Disputed Claims'. I considered six commonly presented claims regarding BSE. These were (1) BSE was caused by sheep material infected with scrapie being fed to cattle. (2) The total number of BSE cases would be 17,000–20,000 in total. (3) The disease is in a dead-end host. (4) It is not possible for BSE to enter the human food chain. (5) The risk of BSE for humans is remote. (6) The number of BSE cases is now dropping. I analysed each claim and found each to be untenable.

35. Later in the year I gave evidence to the European Parliament's Committee of Inquiry into BSE, on 8 October 1996. In my opening remarks I referred to several of my previous publications, including 'Transmissible spongiform encephalopathies: The threat of BSE to man' (see paragraph 16 above), my book *Mad Cow Disease* and 'Bovine Spongiform Encephalopathy – The Disputed Claims' (see paragraph 34 above).

36. On 12 November 1996 I gave the George Orwell Memorial Lecture at Birkbeck College, London, which was published later in the *Political Quarterly* under the title 'The Ministry of Agriculture – the Ministry of Truth'. I endeavoured to illustrate how short-term political interests had taken precedence over national and international risks to human and animal health, by reference to the history of the handling of the BSE crisis.

37. I have written an article to be published in *Reviews in Medical Microbiology* entitled 'Bovine Spongiform Encephalopathy: The Fallout' in which I conclude that measures taken by the UK authorities up to late 1997 are unlikely to prevent BSE from becoming enzootic in a way analogous to sheep scrapie. In my view the number of cases of nv CJD will rise in the next century as a result of direct exposure to bovine material, and it seems likely that intraspecies transfer of nv CJD is expected to occur through, for example, blood materials and surgery, and also by vertical spread.

APPENDIX TWO

Statement by Professor R. W. Lacey

Re: Texas Beef Group, Perryton Feeders Inc., Maltese Cross Cattle Company, Bravo Cattle Company and Alpha 3 Cattle Company.

and

Paul F. Engler and Cactus Feeders, Inc.

v

Oprah Winfrey, Harpo Productions, Inc., Howard Lyman and Cannan Communications, Inc.

I am Richard W. Lacey, and currently hold the posts of Visiting Professor of Medical Microbiology at the University of Leeds, and Consultant Microbiologist to the United Leeds Teaching Hospitals NHS Trust. I am Doctor of Philosophy, Bachelor and Doctor of Medicine (See Appendix I).

Previously I have advised the U.K. Ministry of Agriculture, Fisheries and Food on the use of drugs in animals, fish and birds from 1986–1989. I have been Consultant to The World Health Organisation since 1983. I have researched and published material on the safety of food for at least 10 years, and this has resulted in four general books, each written at the request of publishers (See Appendix I).

My testimony will be organised to comprise a detailed analysis of the section of the Oprah Winfrey programme which is relevant to the plaintiffs case, and then I will comment on the statements by the six experts, in reports submitted on behalf of the plaintiff. The main thrust of my arguments with the latter documents is that substantial parts of these submissions do not actually relate to the complaints.

1   *The claimed offending passages in the Oprah Winfrey programme broadcast on or about 16 April 1996.*

1(a) Winfrey: "You said this disease could make AIDS look like the common cold".

Lyman: "Absolutely".

The analogy between transmissible spongiform encephalopathies (TSEs), of which BSE is one, and AIDS, is highly appropriate. In both types of infection there is a long incubation period when the animal or person is infected, but shows no adverse effects from the presence of the microbe. When the clinical illness does develop, it is slow and progresses to a usual fatal outcome within months or years. Both types of infection, TSEs and HIV, can be passed vertically from an animal dam or the human female to its offspring, and both can be transferred by accident or experiment through the inoculation of infected material into a previously healthy person or animal. Moreover, both these types of infectious diseases are unusual in that their control is difficult because of the long interval when the animal or person is subclinically infected, which can permit often unwittingly, the transfer of the infectious agent to new hosts.

The statement by Ms Winfrey that, "This disease (i.e. BSE) could make AIDS look like the common cold", is an appropriate comment. Over the last few years the annual incidence of AIDS deaths in the U.K. has been around 1,500 per year. Whilst viruses which cause the common cold may cause minor symptoms in the general healthy and ambulatory population, rarely for vulnerable patients, they can be the cause of their death. Certainly, in recent years, more people would have succumbed from AIDS than the common cold, and I have no evidence that these relative effects do not apply to the U.S.A. Ms Winfrey used the verb *could* very accurately. In a leading article (Editorial) in the prestigious International Medical Journal, *The Lancet* of 7 December 1996 (Reference 1), it refers to statements by Professor Adrian Smith, President of the U.K. Royal Statistical Society, that the future number of human Creutzfeldt-Jakob Disease (CJD) cases from BSE could be anything from zero to millions. Later in the article, the

Editor of the journal, Dr Richard Horton (or a person representing his views), confirms that the future number of CJD cases from BSE is, "An estimate that runs from none to several millions". These two views now add to the large number of U.K. scientists who have stated publicly that there *could* be a serious epidemic of CJD due to BSE. Those scientists include myself, Doctor Stephen Dealler, Professor John Patterson and Professor Geofrey Almond.

Thus, Ms Winfrey's statement is, regrettably, correct.

1(b) Lyman: "Absolutely. And what we're looking at – at right now is exactly the same path that they followed in England: 10 years of dealing with it as a public relations exercise rather than doing something about it ......".

This is an accurate assessment of the conduct of the U.K. attitude. The time-scale does extend to 10 years, with first confirmed BSE cases in 1986, and still in 1996 no emphatic eradication measures have been taken, accounting for the persistence of the International ban on U.K. beef products and cattle, including export to the U.S.A. The full details of the public relationship exercise are given in my book; *Mad Cow Disease: the History of BSE in Britain* (Reference 2). The following is a summary of the action taken and it explains how the U.K. population has been exposed to the BSE risk.

I   By mid-late 1987, the following information was known to the Ministry of Agriculture, Fisheries and Food (MAFF). BSE was a new infectious disease of cattle, and it was established that members of the human population were vulnerable to diseases of this sort. Previous research had shown that the infectivity was widely distributed in animals other than cattle that had been either naturally or artificially infected (sheep, goats, mink, rodents, man). Yet it was not until August 1988 that animals with clinical BSE were prohibited from entering the human food chain.

II   Because the vast majority of beef cattle are slaughtered at an age before they show any clinical signs of BSE and there was (and still is) no predictive test, the above prohibition would not be adequate alone to protect the human population from BSE risk. Thus the whole of the animal's carcass (apart from those clinically ill), continued to enter the human food chain from late 1988 to November 1989.

III   In November 1989, six organs were claimed to be now excluded for human consumption from all cattle. These were the specified bovine offals (SBO's) and comprised brain, spinal cord, spleen, thymus, intestines and tonsils. This action was more of a cosmetic attempt at reassurance rather than a genuine attempt to protect the public. It was flawed on four counts:

(i) The delay of its introduction was inexcusable. There had been no relevant new research prior to its implementation.

(ii) Based on the experiments on organs with other species of animals so infected (see above), it is not valid to assume that infectivity in cattle incubating BSE would be confined to those six organs. For example, infectivity in other species had been found by late 1989 in the following organs; nerves, eyes, adrenals, lymph nodes, salivary gland, liver, kidney, lung, uterus, blood and muscle (Reference 7).

(iii) Calves under six months were excluded from the prohibitions. As these diseases were known to be transmissible from the dam to the offspring of other species, by analogy, it should have been anticipated that infectivity could enter the calf at, or before birth.

(iv) Numerous press statements and remarks by the Minister of Agriculture, Mr Douglas Hogg, admitted that spinal cords had not always been removed in the abattoir as late as 1995.

IV   Based on results of feeding experiments, the intestines and thymuses from calves were excluded from the human food chain in June 1994. This clearly indicates that such (and other actions) should have been taken before.

V   At the end of March 1996, the whole of the carcass of cattle aged over 30 months was excluded from the human food chain. This action again is not satisfactory since:

(i) It is often not possible to assess the ages of cattle with accuracy where records are incomplete. The dentition is only a guide.
(ii) It is not known when infectivity for BSE might become dangerous in the animal. There have been 80 cases of BSE in animals whose age has been recorded as less than 30 months.

In summary, the action by MAFF has evidently been a matter of too little, too late, for nearly a decade, and in my opinion Mr Lyman's comments were appropriate.

1(c) Lyman: " ...... One hundred thousand cows per year in the United States are fine at night, dead in the morning ......".

I gather these refer to "Downer" cows, and I have no reason to dispute these numbers, nor do the six experts on behalf of the plaintiffs. Certainly some of the remains of these animals must be expected to be disposed of via the renderers.

1(d) Lyman: "...... The majority of these cows are rounded up, ground up, fed back to other cows ......".

The system of returning unwanted and otherwise unusable cattle remains to cattle feed has been used in many countries for many decades, and is achieved by the inedible remains of cattle, especially old cows, treated in rendering plants, converted to protein extract that is ground up with the bones to yield meat and bone meal that is incorporated into cattle feed by the feed compounders. Although Lyman has abbreviated the process, the statement is accurate.

1(e) Lyman: "...... If only one of them has mad cow disease, it has the potential to infect thousands ......".

This is completely accurate. The word potential in particular is correct. Infectivity of TSEs is measured by the lowest dilution of a tissue slurry that can transmit the disease by experiment. Take the brain for example, of an animal dying of a TSE. This material can be diluted serially ten-fold, by the addition of one gram of brain to nine millilitres (ml) of water, which is then homogenised. This will then produce a one in ten dilution of the brain. This is usually expressed as a dilution of 10^{-1}. When one ml of this diluted brain slurry is added to nine ml of water, the brain is now diluted one in a hundred, or 10^{-2}. The process continues down to a dilution of 10^{-10}. Volumes of these diluted slurries are challenged to a test animal, usually a rodent, and it is quite possible that one ml of a 10^{-8} diluted brain can kill half the mice challenged. This is interpreted to mean that there would be enough infected material to infect 100,000,000 (ie 10^8) mice. Experiments have been performed which have shown that 10,000 target challenged mice can be expected to die from just one gram of BSE brain tissue (Reference 3). This figure is low because the mouse used is not very vulnerable to BSE. But certainly, the claim that one infected cow could infect thousands, is highly plausible. It could however, be millions.

1(f) Lyman: "...... remember 14 per cent of all cows by volume are ground up, turned into feed and fed back to other animals ......".

I cannot comment on the accuracy of this, but it would seem to be compatible with the general activities of the cattle industry, and is not specifically denied by the six expert statements. In general, rendering plants do receive remains of many animals, and the resultant meat and bone meal is used for pigs, sheep, turkeys, chickens, ducks, cattle and many other species.

1(g) Lyman: "We should have them eating grass, not other cows. We've not only turned them into carnivores, we've turned them into cannibals".

The second sentence is accurate and is an interpretation of previous comments. The first sentence is an opinion which I support in principle. Of course, where there is insufficient fresh grass, then silage (stored grass), hay or other cereals can substitute. We must all accept from experience with the Fore tribe in New Guinea (Reference 4) that cannibalism encourages the spread of TSEs. Moreover, the U.K. government banned cattle cannibalism on 18 July 1988.

1(h) Winfrey: "Now doesn't that concern you-all a little bit right here, hearing that? It has just stopped me cold from eating another burger. I'm stopped".

Surely this is a reasonable and natural reaction to an awareness that cattle cannibalism was occurring.

1(i) Lyman: (Next three paragraphs of first amended complain) – page 5. This contains some repetitive material but the following sentence is important.

"...... To-day we should do exactly what the English did and cease feeding cows to cows ......".

This must be obvious common sense. Surely the knowledge of events elsewhere in the world should be reflected in changes in husbandry practices. Some European countries have also taken measures to prevent the spread of BSE by cannibalism, were the disease to enter the system.

1(j) Lyman: "...... Because we have the greedy that are getting the ear of government instead of the needy ......".

Surely this is a very reasonable interpretation of the reason why cattle cannibalism has not ceased in the U.S.A.? I concur with this view.

1(k) Lyman: "...... half the slaughter of - animals is nonsalable to humans".

This is broadly correct.

1(l) Lyman: "...... they grind it up, turn it into something that looks like brown sugar ......".

This is an accurate description of meat and bone meal.

1(m) Lyman: "We ended up feeding downed cows to mink; the mink come down with the disease".

This is true. Transmissible Mink Encephalopathy was considered by researchers to have been due to feeding mink with bovine abattoir waste (Reference 5).

Thus I conclude that all the statements made within the transcript stated to be Exhibit "A" are accurate. It is regrettable that such statements are accurate, and it is inevitable that some members of the public would find these facts repugnant.

I would like to make one further general point. This concerns sporadic Creutzfeldt-Jakob Disease as it occurs in the U.S.A. It is established that this is due to an infectious agent that, apart from medical mishaps, is not transferred between people. Many researchers have considered the likely source of the infection to be animal products (Reference 6) and have excluded sheep scrapie. The most likely source of sporadic CJD is bovine (Reference 7), but this is not capable of being proved nor disproved.

2   *The Evidence of Lester M. Crawford.*

PAGE 1 – Paragraphs 1–3. Nothing relevant to the claims.

PAGE 1 – Paragraph 4.

> "...... Any carcass or meat product shown to be unsafe for human consumption is condemned and diverted from the human food chain ......".

There is no way of identifying whether or not a carcass or meat product is contaminated with BSE under routine conditions.

PAGE 1 – Paragraph 5.

This is a laudable approach, but to prevent the zoonosis BSE, action taken may well have been too late (See below).

PAGE 2 – Paragraph 1 (whole):

It is not clear whether the actual order prohibiting the export of British cattle and bovine by-products, was made in late 1988 or 1989. However, such an action does demonstrate the fear that were BSE to have been introduced into the U.S.A. then the procedures used in the cattle industry would have been such as to enable the disease to spread through cattle cannibalism.

However, this prohibition was too late to be certain to be effective, and is exceedingly unlikely to have been fully implemented for the following reasons.

(a)   Too Late

The first BSE case in the U.K. is now known to have been in late 1985, with the following numbers up to 1994.

Year	No. U.K. confirmed cases MAFF
1985	1
1986	7
1987	420
1988	2,185
1989	7,136
1990	14,180
1991	25,025
1992	35,045
1993	36,755
1994	25,628

Because the average age of death of BSE cases is around 5 years, and the infection is thought to enter the animal around birth (References 2 and 8), then the incubation period is also around 5 years. This means that potentially infected cattle and beef products would have been exported from the U.K. to the U.S.A. between 1981 and late 1988 or early 1989. As seen from the above table, there were about 35,000 BSE cattle confirmed in 1992 and 1993, and these would have in the main acquired the infection in 1987 and 1988. In those years, there were about 1,700,000 cattle of sufficient age to be at risk of developing the disease. This means that about 2% of the U.K. cattle exported from the U.K. to the U.S.A.

would have been expected to have been infected, assuming random relationships between infectivity and export. This is likely to be the case as there was, and still is, no test to identify infected herds before their final illness.

(b) By-products

One of the major cattle by-products is gelatine, extracted from bones of the cow at slaughter. Other sources of gelatine include pig bones, pig skin and cattle skin. When gelatine is used commercially, the detailed sources of its components are often not known. Gelatine is used in a vast array of foods, e.g. ice-cream, yoghurt, sweets, jellies, pies, soups, stocks, mousses and numerous other foods.

In each month of 1996, the U.K. exported about 600 tons of gelatine (data from Angela Browning, Junior Minister of Agriculture, U.K.) and it was not known how much was of a bovine source. Such exported gelatine could go to many countries for production of many types of processed food, which would then enter the U.S.A.

Dr Crawford's claim that 5,000 cattle brains have been examined and BSE has not been found, does not provide reassurance that BSE is not prevalent in the U.S.A. for the following reasons:

(i) The number of studies is too small.
(ii) As far as I am aware, no transmission studies (e.g. to rodents) have been performed
(iii) The changes typical of BSE are very easy to miss in young animals.
(iv) I dispute the claim that rabies suspect cattle represent the population most likely to reveal the presence of BSE in the U.S.A. The most at risk group of cattle for BSE are those aged 4–6 years regardless of whether they are suspected or suffering from rabies.

PAGE 2 – Paragraph 2

From the evidence that I have already submitted, it is likely that BSE is in the U.S.A., but either subclinically (i.e. animals are infected, but there is no diagnostic test, and they appear healthy), or the condition is too rare to be recognised as a specific disease entity.

Dr Crawford's final sentence, "And fairness would dictate that the audience should have been informed that beef by-products are not only consumed by cattle, but by people and virtually all other animals".

Surely the audience does not need to be told that they eat milk, cheese and steak, or their pet dogs or cats do, or pigs or animals in zoos. This is not the issue. Cannibalism has a specific revulsion to people. This is based on well established medical and scientific data, as was shown by the studies on Kuru in the Fore tribe (Reference 4). This revulsion goes back thousands of years and has a similar basis as that to incest. However, Dr Crawford does not deny the occurrence of cattle cannibalism.

PAGE 2 – Paragraph 3, and PAGE 3 – Paragraph 1

I will consider beef sales in Dr Hutcheson's submission.

PAGE 3 – Paragraph 2, and PAGE 4 – Paragraph 1

This contains two relevant statements. The one dealing with temperatures of rendering plants will be considered when assessing Dr Hutcheson's evidence. The other statement as probably made on 14 November 1996 (the date is not fully clear), "BSE now occurs in three countries – the United Kingdom, Switzerland and Portugal", is quite extraordinary for a person who has been asked to submit a statement as an expert witness. BSE has been identified in Northern Ireland, Isle of Man, Jersey, Guernsey, Republic of Ireland, France, Germany, Canada, Italy, Denmark, Oman and the Falkland Islands.

3   *Report by Dr Hutcheson*

In this section, I will refer only to statements not already considered.

PAGE 1 – Paragraph 3

"...... Packing house by products, boning processes, restaurant greases and dead animals are sources of raw materials rendering".

This confirms the occurrence of cattle cannibalism and identifies two further means by which BSE infectivity might enter U.S.A. cattle. These are:

(i) Through the corpses of domestic cats. Over 70 cats in the U.K. have been confirmed as suffering from Feline Spongiform Encephalopathy (FSE), a disease that appears identical in properties to BSE. Cats or other species from the U.K. could therefore introduce the disease to the U.S.A.

(ii) Remains of beef imported into the U.S.A. from the U.K. between 1981 and late 1988 or early 1989 could also have introduced the infectivity to U.S.A. cattle.

PAGE 2 – Paragraph 3

"...... The rendering process takes three to six hours and the raw materials are cooked at 230°F–260°F". (Expressed in Centigrade this range is 110°–127°C).

These temperatures and times are not sufficient to eradicate TSE infectivity. Thus, infectivity of the scrapie agent can survive 160°C (320°F) for 24 hours (Reference 9). The agent responsible for BSE can survive 138°C (280°F) for one hour (Reference 3).

PAGE 2 – Last paragraph, and PAGE 3 (all)

Dr Hutcheson implies that the broadcasting of the Oprah Winfrey Show was responsible for the drop in live cattle prices. However, this would be an example of the well known logical error of *post hoc, ergo hoc*. I do not dispute that the fall in beef prices did occur, and was necessarily related to a drop in beef consumption and demand. However, the fall began on 10 April 1996, six days prior to the Oprah Winfrey broadcast. At this time, beef consumption had dropped dramatically in many parts of the world, particularly in Europe. This was due to the well publicised statement by Stephen Dorrell, U.K. Minister of Health, who on 20 March 1996, stated that there was a possible link between BSE and CJD. This had enormous impact on beef consumption because there was no certain means of identification of the source of beef at the point of its consumption. It was inevitable, in the light of the International trade in beef, that a direct or indirect effect on U.S. beef prices would occur in the weeks following the announcement by Mr Dorrell.

4   *Report by Dr William Hueston*

PAGES 1, 2 and PAGE 3 – Paragraph 1

This describes the surveillance methods used against BSE and admits that there is no certain clinical diagnosis and, "No sensitive and specific live animal test is currently available". Dr Hueston rightly points out the concern over live cattle imported from the U.K. into the U.S.A. between 1980 and 1989. The statement by Dr Hueston at the end of the first paragraph, "By 31 August 1996, brains from a total of 4,816 cattle in the U.S. had been examined neurohistopathologically and no evidence of BSE has been detected", is ambiguous. It is not clear as to whether the figure 4,816 refers to the cattle suspected of rabies, or refers to U.K. cattle, or the total number of brains examined. The figure of 4,816 is certainly similar to the number of rabies suspects mentioned by Dr Crawford (See above).

The great majority of U.K. cattle imported into the U.S.A. between 1980 and 1989 would have been slaughtered by now and their unusable parts rendered and added to cattle feed. Assuming 2% of the U.K. cattle had been infected with BSE in 1987 and 1988, it is difficult to see how this infectivity had not been introduced from U.K. cattle, but still at an incidence or a distribution too low to detect.

PAGE 4 – Paragraph 3

"In March 1996 ......spongiform encephalopathy".

The proposals to end cattle cannibalism because of the, "...... high risk for the potential of transmissible spongiform encephalopathy", would not need to be considered were there confidence about BSE being absent from the U.S. At the time of the Oprah Winfrey programme, this proposal had not been implemented, and this provides the strongest evidence for the defence.

5   *Report by Dr Gary M. Weber*

PAGE 1 – Paragraph 3

"...... Prior to the ban, 499 live cattle imported into the U.S. from the U.K. At this time 39 are known to be alive. Of the original number, more than 40 have been subject to brain analysis. No diagnosis of TSE had been made".

I had previously stated that the incidence of BSE in U.K. cattle rose to a maximum of about 2% in 1987 and 1988. That means that on average, one animal in 50 would be infected. To test the brains of just 40 is therefore not adequate. From these figures I would predict that around 6–8 BSE cattle carcasses (of U.K. origin) would have been rendered and re-fed to a very large number of cattle in the U.S.A. Whilst the infectivity initially might be at too low a concentration to cause disease, the subsequent cycles of cannibalism could provide a very serious epidemic. The experience in the U.K. was that seven BSE cases in 1986 were amplified to over 35,000 in 1992 and 1993.

PAGE 1 – Last sentence

Presumably the date 1985 is incorrect.

6   *Report by Dr R. L. Preston*

This does not provide any specific information, and the points have been considered above.

7   *Report by Fred D. Bisplinghoff and Associates*

PAGE 1 - Four lines from the bottom

" ...... as the BSE agent has never been identified in muscle meat".

This is literally true, but the assays used for the tissue distribution of BSE are unsatisfactory because the breed of mouse challenged is barely vulnerable to BSE. However, equivalent infectivity has been found in the muscles of goats and mink (References 7 and 10).

The claims in the remainder of this submission have been considered previously.

CONCLUSIONS

The statements in the relevant section of the Oprah Winfrey Show, made by herself and Mr Lyman were accurate. The public would have been appalled about the disclosures of cattle cannibalism, but no evidence has been presented that the drop in the auction price of beef, was caused by this programme *per se.*

R. W. Lacey   Date

References

1   Editorial. 'Betraying the public over nv CJD risk'. *Lancet* 1996; 348, 1529.

2   Lacey R. W. *Mad Cow Disease: the History of BSE in Britain*: 1994, Cypsela, St Helier, Jersey.

3   Taylor D. M. *et al.* 'Decontamination studies with the agents of bovine spongiform encephalopathy and scrapie'. *Archives of Virology:* 1994; 139, 313–326.

4   Gajdusek D. C. 'Unconventional viruses and the origin and disappearance of Kuru'. *Science:* 1977; 197, 943–960.

5   Hartsough G. H. and Burger D. 'Encephalopathy of mink. 1. Epizoological and clinical observations'. *Journal of Infectious Diseases:* 1965; 115, 387–392.

6   Davanipour Z. *et al.* 'Transmissible virus dementia: evaluation of a zoonotic hypothesis'. *Neuroepidemiology:* 1986; 5, 194–206.

7   Dealler S. F. and Lacey R. W. 'Transmissible spongiform encephalopathies: The threat of BSE to man'. *Food Microbiology:* 1990; 7, 253–279.

8   Wilesmith J. *et al.* 'Bovine spongiform encephalopathy: epidemiological studies'. *Veterinary Record:* 1988, 123, 638–644.

9   Brown P. *et al.* 'Resistance of scrapie infectivity to steam autoclaving after formaldehyde fixation and limited survival after ashing at 360°C'. *Journal of Infectious Diseases:* 1990; 161, 467–472.

10 Hadlow W. J. *et al.* 'Temporal distribution of transmissible mink encephalopathy virus in mink inoculated subcutaneously'. *Journal of Virology:* 1987; 61, 3235–3240.

APPENDIX THREE

Transmissible spongiform encephalopathies: The threat of BSE to man

Stephen F. Dealler and Richard W. Lacey
Department of Microbiology, University of Leeds, Leeds LS2 9JT, UK.

(This article was first published in Food Microbiology, 7 (1990) pp. 253–79.)

Transmissible spongiform encephalopathies in mammals (TSEs) are due to ultra-filtrable agents of prodigious resistance to physical agents. The exact nature of the infectious agent is not known, possibly being a virus-like (virino) structure or a proteinaceous agent (prion). Some of the proteins found in tissues from infected animals may result from the host response to the infectious agents. The resultant diseases are slowly developing dementias and paralyses, although the infective agent is found in many tissues. The route of acquisition is thought to be mainly through ingestion, with some evidence of vertical transmission. The host range of each agent is modified unpredictably by passage in a new species. The infective agent responsible for Bovine Spongiform Encephalopathy (BSE) was acquired through incorporation of animal products into cattle feed. The source of this product has not been identified, nor has its host range. There is a distinct possibility that man could acquire spongiform encephalopathy from consumption of contaminated beef.

Introduction

Transmissible spongiform encephalopathy (TSE) is an accurate description of a group of inevitably fatal diseases in several mammals. Those said to be naturally affected include sheep, man, cattle, mink, deer and cats. It is debatable whether the mode of acquisition of bovine spongiform encephalopathy (BSE) by cattle, kuru by man, and spongiform encephalopathy (SE) by cats is in reality 'natural'. The disease does seem to be confined to mammals, and both the clinical features and the understanding of the nature of the presumed infective agents justifies the placing of these into one group. The clinical features result from slowly developing alterations and destruction of neurons. Although these diseases are primarily seen as brain diseases, the infective agents have been found in many tissues (*vide infra*).

The timescale of the disease in each species is characteristic: there is a long incubation period, usually of some years, followed by a progressive sub-acute illness over many weeks or months.

In most cases, three cellular changes are evident in brain material from infected animals. These are a degeneration of neurones, the cells actually responsible for brain function, a hypertrophy or enlargement of the supporting astrocytes, and a diffuse sponge-like appearance sometimes referred to as status spongiosus. In some cases the diagnosis is not clear cut and there are problems in distinguishing TSE from other diseases (Zlotnik and Rennie 1965, Hadlow et al. 1982, Collinge et al. 1990). The clinical pictures of the disease can also be variable. These two factors contribute to some of the uncertainties over the actual incidence of TSEs.

Scrapie in sheep has been the TSE most studied in animals. It was first described with confidence by Leopold in 1759 in Germany. This disease is found in many countries, including Britain and France and the incidence is said to be high in Iceland, and exceedingly low in New Zealand. Caution must be made in accepting some estimates of the incidence of scrapie because of the shortcomings in procedures for recording cases. Sigurdsson (1954) made the important observation that after eradication of the whole sheep population in the area where the disease is endemic in Iceland, scrapie appeared a few years later in the new flocks which were imported from a region where scrapie had never existed, with the same annual loss as before eventually. This does raise the possibility that the new flocks were infected from residual agents on the ground which has some disturbing implications for the long term elimination of BSE from cattle.

Scrapie generally presents as one of two clinical types, although the features can overlap. In the scratching form, there can be frenzied rubbing of the back legs by the head or scraping the body against walls, posts or trees. The animal is often weak, tending to fall easily. It shows enhanced fear to stimuli. In the other type, the infected sheep shows stubborn reactions to stimuli, jerky movements of limbs or ears or stretching back of the head. The muscles may visibly tremble (fasciculation) and the gait may resemble that of a donkey ('cuddly trot'). Sometimes an extreme thirst sets in. By the time that the symptoms are advanced, the animal is destroyed. Scrapie appears to have been prevalent in the UK since the eighteenth century (Critchley et al. 1972).

As will be discussed below, the remarkable observation is that BSE did not appear in cattle on a major scale until the last few years despite sheep and cattle sharing the same pastures for centuries. Any hypothesis on the aetiology of BSE must account for this. One of the human TSEs, Creutzfeldt-Jakob disease (CJD), was described independently by these two authors (Creutzfeldt 1921, Jakob 1921). It was first known as 'spastic pseudosclerosis' or 'subacute spongiform encephalopathy' and various other workers' names have been associated with disease. The illness occurs mainly sporadically, although a familial incidence is described in about 15% of cases. Most cases occur in late middle age (50–60 years) in both sexes. Some younger people have been afflicted, although the confidence with which the diagnosis is made varies. There is an understandable reluctance for some pathologists to perform post-mortem examinations on patients thought to have succumbed from CJD (Critchley et al. 1972, Report 1981).

The first symptoms are pains and trembling in muscles, and loss of coordination (particularly in walking) may occur. Uncontrolled twitching of the eyes (nystagmus) and tremors are common. Double vision, difficulty in speaking, and muscles spasticity are often seen. Mental changes include depression, loss of memory and confusion. Blindness and epilepsy are frequent. Towards the end of the illness, the patient is confined to bed, is incontinent, helpless, and requires constant nursing. Death usually occurs between 3 and 9 months after the onset of the illness. However, this can vary from a few weeks to 5 years.

Another human TSE, kuru, occurred in the Fore tribe, a stone-age civilisation in the remote highlands of New Guinea. The disease kuru was prevalent during the first half of this century. Most authorities have attributed cannibalism, notably eating brain, as the cause of the disease, although it is possible that the infective agent can enter the body through cuts of the skin while handling brains in funeral rituals. As with CJD, the clinical picture of the disease involves progressive damage to musculo-skeletal functions and those of intellect.

The disease is now rarer, as a result of education. Before the 1950s, women, who were mostly involved with cannibalism, predominantly suffered from the disease. The age at which the illness typically developed was often between 20 and 40 (e.g. Critchley et al. 1972).

The relationship between the potential for infectivity of the host through oral ingestion with findings from experimentally induced infection through intracerebral inoculation requires clarification. Thus, if an agent generates an infection through intracerebral inoculation, it may not do so necessarily orally or, if it does, the incubation period may be longer. Similarly, the failure to establish an infection intracerebrally in a few animals of a species cannot be taken to assume that every member would resist oral challenge.

BSE: Clinical and statistical aspects
Because of their generally greater longevity, most cases of BSE have been reported in cows rather than cattle. A good description of the clinical disease comes from a farm that has had a large number of cases (Winter et al. 1989). Initially, the cow appears mentally alert, but unusually anxious and apprehensive. It takes a wide base stance, and the abdomen is drawn up. The gait becomes abnormal and exaggerated, and the animal splays its hind limbs when turning sharply, especially on wet surfaces, which gives rise to tumbling and skin wounds. Appetite is the same as unaffected cows but faeces are firmer. However, the animal loses weight and produces less milk. Fine muscle fasciculations involving small muscle groups over the surface of the neck and body are seen and occasionally myoclonic (i.e. repetitive and vigorous jerks) occur (Hope et al. 1989, Scott et al. 1989). The tone of the 'moo' can change and apparently aimless head butting is seen with other anxious and frenzied movements.

Changes are seen in the electroencephalopath pattern of the cow's brain activity and also in the CSF chemistry (Scott et al. 1990) but no antibodies specific to the disease are produced and no specific tests are available while the animal is alive, except of course unpracticable brain biopsy.

Claims have been made that this is not a new disease, it having been seen in approximately one cow in 20 000–30 000 in the past (Eddy 1990b). Similar clinical symptoms can be seen with other conditions (e.g.

Table 1. The age of cows (when available) at time of slaughter due to BSE in England and Wales in 1989 (Hansard 1990g).

Age (years)	Number of cases
1–2	1[a]
2–3	28
3–4	586
4–5	2138
5–6	1874
6–7	667
7–8	125
8–9	37
9–10	8
10–11	3
11–12	1
12–13	1
15–16	1

[a]22 months

magnesium deficiency), but these respond to treatment and are generally not fatal. The discussion as to whether it is a new disease has continued (Marr 1990) and it has been claimed that the condition previously had a different name (P. Hayes, pers. commun.) being called 'stoddy' in Yorkshire.

BSE was first comprehensively documented in the UK in 1986, and the British Isles remain the only certain source, although two calves were exported to Oman that subsequently developed the illness (Carolan et al. 1990). The disease infects Holstein Friesian breed milking cows and other breeds. There is little reason to believe that any one breed is particularly susceptible although, as with many infections, a genetic predisposition may occur among individual animals (Wijeratne and Curnour, 1990).

Epidemiology suggests (Editorial 1988, Southwood 1989) that BSE initially infected animals from 1981/2 and that the majority of animals became infected in calfhood (Wilesmith et al. 1988) through their food (Morgan 1988), giving an incubation period of approximately 3–6 years (Table 1). The continuation of this mode of infection of cows should have stopped following the prevention of rendered mammalian tissue being incorporated in cattle food in 1988. Some veterinarians are fearful that the disease will be passed from the cow to the calf and hence may not be eradicated (Tyrell 1989, Aldhouse 1990, Grant 1990), whereas the British

Parliamentary Agricultural Committee does not share this worry (Report 1990). It is also possible theoretically that the capacity of the infectious agent to survive rigorous environmental extremes (*vide infra*) will enable it to persist on grassland and infect new generations of cattle.

Relatively few cases have been reported from Scotland, Northern Ireland or the Republic of Ireland. The distribution in England and Wales is shown in Fig. 1 (see page 269) (Hansard 1990e). Apparently no cases have been reported from the Isle of Man. On 15 February 1990 the largest number of cases of BSE on a farm was 29, the average number in an infected herd was 1.75, the proportion of herds with a single case was 63%, the proportion of all dairy herds that have had at least one case was 10%, and 0.7% of all beef herds have had one or more cases (Hansard 1990b). The concentration of cases in the South of England means that these figures can only be a guide. For instance, the annual incidence of BSE in the total population of adult cattle in the UK is 0.2% but a veterinarian in the South of England may ultimately see 10% of the dairy cows on large local farms with the disease (M. Winter, pers. commun.).

It should not be forgotten that bulls with BSE have been reported (Hansard 1990c), that Scotland may have low numbers but is also affected (Hansard 1990h), and that the mounting compensation costs to the Government are not small [more than 6 million pounds to February 1990 (Hansard 1990f)].

Diagnostic methods for BSE are developing rapidly through PrP detection techniques (*vide infra*) (Hope et al. 1988, Farquhar et al. 1989) but currently histological examination of brain tissue is used for this purpose. Currently we do not know the percentage of cattle that are being slaughtered that are infected with BSE (Hansard 1990a) and research into this has not been undertaken (Tyrrell 1989, Southwood 1989). We do not know the time at which the animal becomes infective during the incubation of the disease and we do not know how it is passed, or to which animals it will cause disease.

History of BSE
The numbers of cows reported to the British Government with BSE is shown in Table 2 (Hansard 1990e, g).

BSE was first reported by the technical staff at the Central Veterinary Laboratory, Weybridge, Surrey, in November 1986 (Tyrrell 1989). The

Table 2. Cumulative number of cases of BSE reported per year in England and Wales.

Year	Number of cases
1986	7
1987	413
1988	2247
1989	6420
1990	17434[a]

[a] Estimated from figures to April 1990 (Hansard 1990e, g). However, by the end of June 1990, nearly 20 000 cases had been reported, suggesting that the total for 1990 will be around 25 000.

small initial numbers of reported cases quickly increased as more farmers realised the relevance of neurological symptoms in cows on their farm. It is probable that an apparent BSE epidemic arose because large numbers of cows were being fed a protein supplement which contained the brain tissue or other offals of animals (possibly other cows or sheep) that were suffering from either scrapie or from other TSE (Tyrrell 1989, Report 1990). The British Government banned the use of ruminant tissue in food supplements to cows in July 1988 (Report 1990) but the same animal food could still be exported to Europe despite widespread demands that this should not happen (Hansard 1989). This may have led to large numbers of cattle in Europe being infected (Horizon 1990), although it is likely that few will have already shown signs of disease. Also in July 1988, the British Government introduced legislation demanding compulsory reporting of animals that are considered to have BSE, compulsory slaughter and compensation to the farmer at 50% of the market value and disposal of their meat and milk (Report 1990). The rapid rise in numbers of affected cows, particularly in the South of England (Southwood 1989, Hansard 1990g), gave rise to increasing interest from the press and, when the report of the Working Party of Bovine Spongiform Encephalopathy (the 'Southwood' Report) appeared in January 1989, the public interest in the condition increased dramatically.

The relative paucity of infected animals in Scotland has not been explained by published information. Presumably, the degree of contamination of the feed by disease-inducing material varies with product. Details of this are presumably available to MAFF, but not to the authors of this article! One possible factor may have been the need to use protein supplements where the availability of grass and silage was least. The climate in Southern England could therefore have been a decisive factor.

The Southwood Report recommended that a second committee should look into the research that was needed to investigate BSE: The Consultative Committee on Research into Spongiform Encephalopathies (the 'Tyrrell' Committee). This committee, soon after its initiation, asked the British Government to ban all bovine tissues that had been shown in other species to be infective for SE (the gut, lymphoid and nervous tissues) from human consumption. This was announced in June 1989 but not enacted until November 1989 and this gap allowed the potentially infected nervous, gut and lyphoid tissue of approximately 2 million cattle to reach human food. The report of this committee was submitted to the government in June 1989 but not published until January 1990 (Tyrrell 1989).

By June 1989, 150 cows a week were being reported as having BSE. When the amount of compensation was raised to the full sale price of the cow in February 1990, the numbers of cows reported with BSE initially rose by a further 73% (Hansard 1990i). Hence, it is likely that prior to this many of the cows with BSE were not being notified.

The report of an SE in a five-year-old male Siamese cat in May 1990 (Wyatt et al. 1990) and the further reports of SE in zoo animals (Gibson 1990, Hansard 1990d) brought into doubt the main credence in the 'Southwood' report that BSE was not a threat to man. It had been hoped that the cow would be a 'dead end' host for BSE as there was no evidence that it would be transmitted to other hosts. However, there appeared to be few resources other than BSE that could have infected the cat and reports of further cases have followed this. The possibility that Southwood was not correct and that the beef was infective was taken up by the media and the demand for beef slumped.

The demands by the French and German governments (although many other European Governments were also involved) in May 1990 that British beef should not be imported to their countries led to the agreement that only beef from farms that had no history of BSE (specifically, no clinical case within the previous 2 years) would be exported to them. At the current time the auction price of a cow for slaughter from a BSE free herd is 142% that from a herd with BSE. That the value of a cow from a herd with a history of BSE is much lower than one from a BSE free herd means it is very much against the farmer's interest to report a new case.

The media activity, the loss of profits of farmers and the difficulties within the European Community led the House of Commons Agriculture Committee to produce a report on BSE in July 1990. The report declared that British beef was safe to eat, but questioned the activity in abattoirs of splitting bovine heads to remove the brain, the breeding of cattle that may be infected with BSE, and the inclusion of potentially infected meat in pet food. The report also asked that calves also be included in the ban on brain and lymphoid tissue being taken for human consumption, and it asked that mechanically recovered meat and the use of saws in the cutting of animal carcasses that may be infected be stopped (Report 1990). In the evidence of this committee, Tyrrell stated that he expected that one in a thousand cows that came to slaughter for human consumption should be considered infected (Report 1990). The tight measures to control BSE are expected to revive the demand for British beef. However, further announcements in the veterinary press concerning the infectivity of the meat of scrapie infected goats (Pattison 1990), the possibility of infection being passed accidentally between cows by needle injection or by surgical procedure (Lees 1990), may have blunted this hope.

By May 1990 the number of reported cases had reached around 300–400 per week; higher than the ability of the Ministry of Agriculture Fisheries and Food (MAFF) to dispose of the carcasses by incineration. Animals have been reported having been dumped into open waste sites for disposal (Keighley News 1990). This practice is apparently within current legislation.

British farmers now declare that beef farming is not profitable at current prices (which have dropped by approximately 20%), but despite this land prices have stayed steady and farmers are moving into other produce. The increased cost of cows and their offspring being registered in order to prevent the calves of infected cows being used for mating may be born by the Government but beef farming is currently uneconomic despite this.

The suggestion that cases of BSE have appeared in France and in the United States (Horizon 1990) have not been confirmed in the scientific literature. However, the continuing practice of feeding animal protein to cows in European countries may represent a threat. The export from Britain of calves which may be infected with BSE raises the possibility of similar epidemics in other countries.

Epidemiology of TSE in other animals

It has been established that scrapie can be transmitted between sheep within the same flock, that lambs of an infected ewe were more likely to become ill than those of an uninfected one, and that sheep that had grazed on land that had previously supported sheep with scrapie also might acquire the disease. Some sheep seemed to develop scrapie spontaneously, with no contact with infected animals.

The disease can be transferred by injection of brain material from an infected to an uninfected animal. Subsequently, much of the experimental work has been performed in laboratory animals, such as hamsters and mice on account of their short incubation periods (often less than 1 year). However, in passaging the scrapie agent to different species, the incubation period can increase, the histopathology changes, and the infected animal shows atypical clinical signs (Pattison 1988). This has been termed the 'species barrier'. Moreover, once the infection was passed into a different species, there was also a 'species barrier' in attempts to pass the disease back to the original donor species. When passed onto another animal of the same species, however, the incubation period decreased, and the histopathology became the same as with further generation infections, as did the clinical signs. These findings suggest that passage through a new mammalian species changes the properties of the infective agent.

Such transfer of TSE has been achieved by intracerebral injection (Kimberlin and Walker 1979), percutaneously (Eklund et al. 1967, Kimberlin and Walker 1979, Matthews 1981), intraperitoneally (Kimberlin et al. 1971), intraocularly (Kimberlin and Walker 1986), intragastrically (Kimberlin and Walker 1989), intranervously (Field and Hill 1974, Fraser 1982) and through injections of infected tissue. Unfortunately this happened by accident due to the contamination of louping ill vaccine with scrapie (Brotherston et al. 1968) and concern has been proposed about the possible contamination of human growth hormone derived from human pituitary (Report 1990).

One animal ingesting infected material derived from another has been considered to be the cause of infection when different animals are kept in the same cage and the disease is passed between them, e.g. mice (Pattison 1964) and mink (Hadlow et al. 1987). This was thought to be due to bites or scratches of one animal by another as it might occur between two animals in adjacent cages (this work has yet to be confirmed).

Disease transfer has been presumed to be oral in the natural state in sheep (Pattison and Millson 1961, Pattison et al. 1972) and the newborn lamb has not been shown to be infected, but the placenta is (Hadlow et al. 1982). Scrapie can be produced in a sheep by feeding the foetal membranes of an infected animal (Pattison et al. 1974) and this is a favoured method by which scrapie is thought to pass to offspring. The placenta is often eaten by the ewe. The contamination of the pasture and the resilience of the infective agent have meant that this has been thought to be the method of lateral transfer between sheep (Pattison 1964, Morgan 1988) although this has been disputed (Wilson et al. 1950). It has also been suggested that contact is all that is required to transfer scrapie between animals (Brotherston et al. 1968).

Oral transmission of TSEs has been achieved with scrapie in sheep (Pattison et al. 1972), mice (Carp 1982, Kimberlin and Walker 1989), goats (Pattison and Millson 1962), hamsters (Prusiner et al. 1985) and mink (Hanson et al. 1971). Transmissible mink encephalopathy has been transmitted orally to mink (Burgher and Hartsough 1965), CJD to squirrel monkeys (Matthews 1981) and BSE to mice. The full scope of the potential for the oral route of transfer of TSEs between mammals is not yet established. The scarification of the gums may change the likelihood of passing the TSE by mouth (Carp 1982), but it is clear that it can pass orally between species without this.

Effect of host passage on the properties of the infectious agent
Attempts to produce prion infections (*vide infra*) in animals have not always been successful. Some animals appear to be more vulnerable than others and some laboratory strains seem to possess variations in susceptibility so that only a proportion of the animals when given what was anticipated to be an infective dose actually develop the disease.

Strain variation as shown by alteration in general biological properties has been seen in scrapie (*vide supra*). Propagation of such agents on a new

Table 3. Range of animals to which SE from various animals can be transmitted (see text; in particular Prusiner 1984, Davanipour et al. 1986, Hope et al. 1989, Dawson et al. 1990)

Host	CJD	Scrapie[a]	TME	Kuru	Cow
Human	+	NT	NT	NT	NT
Sheep	–	+	+	–	NT
Mink	–	+	+	–	+[b]
Cow	NT	+	–	NT	+
Chimpanzee	+	–	–	+	NT
Gibbon	–	–	–	+	NT
New-world monkey					
Capuchin	+	–	NT	+	NT
Marmoset	+	NT	NT	+	NT
Spider					
Squirrel	+	+	+	+	NT
Woolly	+	NT	NT	+	NT
Old-world monkey					
Cynomolgus	–	+	NT	–	NT
Managabey	+	NT	NT	–	NT
Rhesus	–	–	+	+	NT
Pig-tailed	+	NT	NT	+	NT
Bonnet	NT	NT	NT	+	NT
African green	+	–	NT	–	NT
Baboon	+	NT	NT	NT	NT
Bush baby	+	NT	NT	–	NT
Patas	+	NT	NT	NT	NT
Stump-tailed	–	NT	+	–	NT
Talapoin	+	NT	NT	NT	NT
Goat	+	+	+	–	NT
Ferret (albino)	+?	NT	+	NT	NT
Cat	+	NT	–	–	+[c]
Racoon	NT	NT	+	NT	NT
Skunk	NT	NT	+	NT	NT
Mouse	+	+	–	–	+
Rat	–	+	NT	–	NT
Hamster (golden)	+	+	+	–	–[d]
Gerbil	+	–	NT	–	NT
Vole	NT	+	NT	NT	NT
Guinea-pig	+	–	+	–	NT
Rabbit	–	–	–	–	NT
Pig	NT	NT	NT	NT	+

[a] Various primates inoculated with mouse adopted scrapie failed to develop the disease.
[b] Presumed from outbreak of TME at Stetsonville, USA.
[c] Presumed from epidemiology experimental work to follow.
[d] Current findings at Central Veterinary Laboratory.
+ denotes transfer of infectious agent.
NT, not tested.
NB: relatively little work has been done on chronic wasting disease of deer, which can be transmitted to the ferret. The British zoological animals: kudu, oryx, nyala, gemsbok and eland have also acquired SE but the origin is unknown.

host could well modify the agent's potential infectivity for other hosts. This results from the possible incorporation of host cellular material in the surface of the particle. Transmissible mink encephalopathy (TME) is thought by some to have been derived from scrapie, and yet its host range differs from that of scrapie (Davanipour et al. 1986) (Table 3).

It follows from this that even if it is assumed that scrapie did transfer to cattle as BSE, and the scrapie agent in sheep was not infectious to man, it is not possible to exclude the possibility that the BSE agent from cattle is infectious to man.

Approximately 50% of the animal species that have been inoculated or fed with the agents responsible for scrapie, CJD, TME and kuru have been shown to become infected subsequently (See Table 3) (Davanipour et al. 1986). This has occurred through a variety of routes, but that each of the 'natural' encephalopathies has a different range of infection to any other species suggests that we should assume that BSE has a characteristic and a large undefined host range specificity. Thus, TME is thought to have been derived from the feeding of scrapie to mink (Burgher and Hartsough 1965, Hartsough and Burgher 1965, Hanson et al. 1971, Hadlow et al. 1987) but it has a clearly different range of infectivity. In particular, the agent from sheep has no affinity for rhesus monkeys but that from mink has (Hanson et al. 1971). The species barrier has been shown much more clearly in rats by Pattison and Jones (1968), where strain types of 'scrapie' infecting the rats changed after infecting them. The recent reports of a feline spongiform encephalopathy (FSE) (Wyatt et al. 1990) may indicate that BSE may have infected cats (Report 1990). Scrapie infected meat has been fed to cats for many years and there have been no reports of FSE. Similar reports of novel SEs in zoo animals such as antelopes (Gibson 1990) are highly relevant. The alternative proposal that FSE and encephalopathies in zoo animals are not truly novel, but just newly recognised cannot be ruled out, but seems most unlikely. We must assume that the agent causing BSE will have a different associated proteinacious structure from that of the agent causing scrapie (Endo et al. 1989, Goldman et al. 1990); it will also have a different range of infectivity in the same way as the causative agent of TME. The possibility that BSE was derived not from scrapie but from another SE would also be consistent with this. BSE may well have been due to the feeding of offal derived from a cow which was suffering from a sporadic case of SE to other cows, and then the feeding of their tissues to further animals. At each passage this would multiply the infectivity of the feed.

If BSE follows the general potential of the TSEs to infect about 50% of other mammalian species, then those with responsibility for control of infection should assume that humans are included until this is proved not to be the case. The prion chemistry of sporadic cases of CJD are apparently the same and this may suggest that they are not sporadic mutants but true infections. This is considered in more detail below. There are few animals that we eat which live long enough to become infective with SE. The possibility that CJD represents human infections with the previous rare sporadic or subclinical cases of BSE has not been investigated but would suggest that human beings are at risk of catching BSE orally from infected bovine tissues. There appears to be little association between the incidence of scrapie in sheep and CJD (Southwood 1989). Pig products are generally consumed from animals less than 6 months old. The only other mammals commonly consumed at an age for such an infectious agent to be present in large amounts are cows and cattle.

Infective tissue from TSE infected animals

To find out which tissues from an animal suffering from SE are infective is very expensive and time consuming. Small amounts of tissue from the infected animal are injected intracerebrally into an animal strain that is known to be vulnerable to infection. This can be done at different points during the progress of infected animals' disease in order to find out at what point the tissue becomes infective, or may be done when the animal shows clinical signs of infection. Neither of these processes has been carried out systematically for BSE but they are planned (Tyrrell 1989). Hence, in the absence of any contrary data it should be assumed that BSE is similar to SE in other animals (see Tables 4 and 5).

These figures may give an impression of every type of tissue that has been tested being found to be infected. Indeed, the low sensitivity [often 10^3 infective units (IU) per gram of tissue] of the test technique used by some researchers may mean that these are underestimates of the infectivity of the tissues. However, the relevance of these to the possibility of human infection via the oral route must be cautioned. Many researchers have not been able to reproduce other work in showing the infectivity of some tissues (Eklund et al. 1967, Pattison et al. 1972, Hadlow et al. 1974, Casaccia et al. 1989). Thus meat, blood, milk, faeces and urine are considered either not infective at all or to a relatively low degree (Eklund et al. 1967, Pattison et al. 1972, Hadlow et al. 1974). However, in the abattoir it is difficult to stop nervous or lymphoid tissue being present in meat for human consumption (Report 1990). Approximately one in five cattle that go to slaughter for human consumption are dairy cattle, and hence at greatest risk of being infected with BSE. It is unclear which tissues of these animals should be considered potentially infective to humans.

Infective period of animals with a spongiform encephalopathy

The infective units (IU) are first found in the spleen and lymphoid tissue of the animal that has been infected (Table 4) (Eklund et al. 1967, Hadlow et al. 1974), and this is followed by increasing numbers of infection-generating particles in nervous tissue (Eklund et al. 1967, Hadlow et al. 1974). It has been claimed that peripheral nerves carry the infective agent towards the central nervous system and that the spinal cord becomes infected before the brain (Kimberlin and Walker 1979, 1986, 1989). The spleen starts to contain IU soon after intravenous injection of infective material in the animal (Eklund et al. 1967). This is also shown with local injection into the gastric wall (Kimberlin and Walker 1989). Other tissues become infective more slowly and it is probable that lymphoid tissue, all abdominal organs, and nervous tissue become infective between one-half and two-thirds of the duration of the incubation period. Therefore, it is clear that clinically well cattle might contain the infectious agent, and this is obviously important with respect to food safety (vide infra).

The experiments with SE in many species have the problem of the delay before intracerebrally injected animals show signs of disease. This may be as little as 3 months in mice or it may be 5 years in larger mammals, depending on the species. When SE passes from one species to another the incubation period can increase (Pattison and Millson 1961, Zlotnik and Rennie 1965, Pattison and Jones 1968, Hanson et al. 1971, Kimberlin and Marsh 1975, Kimberlin and Walker 1979, Hadlow et al. 1987). For primates this may be many years but experimenters cannot be expected to wait 20 years to find out if an infection has taken place and this may make the experiments difficult with BSE.

Table 4. Stage of incubation period at which tissues were first found to be infectious. (See Pattison and Millson 1961, 1962, Marsh et al. 1967, Eklund et al. 1967, Hadlow et al. 1974, 1987)

Tissue	\% of incubation period								
	30	40	50	60	70	80	90	100[b]	110
Brain				m,g, mk					
Pituitary					g				
Spinal cord		m		g,mk					
Peripheral nerve					g,mk				
Spleen	m[a]	g				mk			
Adrenal					g				
Lymph node	g,mk								
Thymus	m[a],mk								
Lung		m							
Liver/kidney						mk		m	
Muscle									g
Gut	m,g							mk	
Bone marrow						m			
Salivary gland				g		mk			

[a] Infectivity started at 14% of incubation period.
[b] 100% incubation period coincides with onset of clinical disease.
m, g and mk represent the incubation period percentage at which the tissue infective in mice, goats and mink.

Human kuru may sometimes have an incubation time of more than 30 years and this may represent the low number of infective particles that gain access to the nervous system as the incubation period is also inversely related to the infecting dose (Pattison and Millson 1961, Kimberlin and Walker 1978, Prusiner 1980, 1982, 1984). Because *Homo sapiens* lives so long, we may be open to infection by relatively low numbers of IU.

Destruction of the agent

Most disinfectant chemicals (e.g. domestic bleach) do not appear to neutralise the infectivity of the agent (Taylor 1989), and neither do proteinases (specifically those found in the animal gut, Prusiner 1984), DNAase (Pattison 1988), RNAase (Prusiner 1984), ultraviolet light (Prusiner 1982), ionising irradiation at usable doses (Fraser et al. 1989), or heat (cooking temperatures) (Dickinson and Taylor 1978). Protease K has been shown to decrease infectivity as have specific chemicals that react with protein (Prusiner 1984). However, the chemicals that react specifically with DNA or RNA (psoralen photoadducts, hydroxylamine)

Table 5. Tissues found to be infected by their ability to infect further animals

Tissue	Sheep	Goat	Mouse	Mink	Man	Cow
			Animal[a]			
Brain	+	+	+	+	+	+
Spinal cord	+	+	+	+	+	
Peripheral nerve	+	+	+			
Eye					+	
Adrenal		+				
Lymph node	+	+	+	+		
Tonsil		+				
Salivary gland	–	+	+	+		
Spleen	+	+	+	+	+	
Gut	+	+	+	+		
Liver		+	+	+		
Kidney	–	–	+	+		
Bladder				+		
Pancreas		–				
Heart	–	–				
Lung	–	–	+	+		
Thyroid	–					
Thymus			+	+		
Testis		–				
Ovary		–				
Uterus			+			
Blood/serum	–	–	–	+	+	
Bone marrow		–	+	–		
CSF	–	+			+	
Urine	–			–	–	
Faeces				+	–	
Saliva	–	–			–	
Milk	–					
Muscle[b]	–	+		+		
Mammary gland	–					

[a] Sheep (Hadlow et al. 1982); goat (Pattison and Millson 1962, Hadlow et al. 1974); mouse (Pattison and Jones 1968); mink (Hadlow et al. 1987, Marsh et al. 1969); man (Matthews 1981); cow (Hope et al. 1988).

[b] Scrapie infected hamsters also have infective muscle tissue.

do not have any affect (Prusiner 1984). Autoclaving at 134°C for 1 h decreases the infectivity of CJD or scrapie material to low levels (Rohiner 1984) but there is still evidence that full destruction has not taken place. Some infectivity of the scrapie agent can survive baking for 24 h at 160°C in dry heat (Taylor 1989) or at 360°C for 1 h (Brown et al. 1990). The only ways of ensuring destruction of these agents are with concentrated (e.g. normal) mineral alkalis.

The American current standard for autoclaving for decontamination of CJD is 132°C for 1 h (Rosenberg 1986). In Britain several methods are recommended for decontamination; the most common one used is 136–138°C for 18 min (Report 1981). This is aimed to prevent the transfer of the infective agent for CJD between patients by metal electrodes, corneal transplants (Behan 1982), dental procedures (Adams and Edgar 1978), or in the laboratory (Manuelidis et al. 1985, Miller 1988). Pathologists are often unwilling to undertake postmortem examinations of patients considered as possibly having died of CJD and when they do, gloves, autoclaving gowns and cap, over-shoes, and masks are worn along with a disposable plastic apron under the operation gown (Report 1981).

The MAFF sent out 'Guidance for veterinary surgeons handling known or suspected cases of BSE' to all District Veterinary Officers giving directions as to how to deal with cows that are thought to be infected with BSE. This did not state, however, that many cows that showed no sign of the illness might be infected and therefore a possible risk to other mammals, including man. As an example of this, in 1989 14 cases of BSE occurred in a herd in Surrey. In 1990 there were 60–80 (Winter, pers commun.), suggesting the probable existence of 46–66 infected animals that remained undetected in 1989. The British Veterinary Association recommended to its members that, contrary to the MAFF's suggestions, no veterinarians should take part in calving or caesarian sections of infected cows (Cooke 1990, Editorial 1990).

Abattoir workers and farmers have been treated in a different light in that animals have been split open mechanically and sawn using circular saws, animals have had their heads removed to be sent to MAFF in Weybridge, Surrey, and headless cows have been carried in blood-dripping lorries to sites of incineration. Farmers have not been warned about the possible danger of infective products to other cows (or to themselves) during calving, killing or eating of an infected animal. In large farms in parts of the South of England, BSE is now reaching 10% of the dairy stock and abattoir workers have not been warned as doctors or veterinary surgeons have.

Chemical structure of TSE infective agents
The two main structures that are considered the likely candidates for the actual infectious agent are the virino and the prion (Prusiner 1982).

(1) Virino

This is made up of a small fragment of DNA associated with the proteinase material (Kimberlin 1982, Prusiner 1982, Collinge et al. 1989, Southwood 1989). The DNA would be involved in induction of the protein from the DNA of the brain. However, no DNA has been found associated with the infective fragments (except by Narang et al. 1988), and DNAase, psoralens and amidines (Prusiner 1984) do not decrease its infectivity, nor does ionising radiation (Fraser et al. 1989).

(2) Prion (see Prusiner 1989)

This is a sialoglycoprotein derived from the DNA of the infected cell but which is changed by the infecting particle. This protein has been isolated from infected species and evidence for its role is mounting. The major problem with this hypothesis is its inability to account for variation among the different strains of scrapie. Some of these variants infect some species that others cannot. There is also variation in the length of incubation periods. It is not clear how such variation can be generated if the infecting particle was derived from the DNA of the host genome (Pattison 1988).

The argument that the infective particle must contain its own DNA particle (Kimberlin 1982, Manuelidis 1985, Prusiner 1989) or need not (Kimberlin 1982, Prusiner et al. 1983, Bockman et al. 1985, Braig and Diringer 1985, Basler et al. 1986, Gabizon et al. 1988), continues.

The chemical structures of the virino and prion are well reviewed by Prusiner (1989), Manuelidis (1985), and Griffin (1985).

Scrapie associated fibrils (SAF) and prion rods are found by electron microscopy only in the brain of SE infected animals, and the PrP (prion protein) is found in all animals with SE disease but is produced by the genes of the host animal. After concentration these can be studied microscopically and chemically.

Concentration of infectivity from scrapie infected tissue

This can initially be carried out using molecular properties, partial purification and assay of the tissue using hamsters (Prusiner 1980, Manuelidis et al. 1987, Sklaviadis et al. 1989). In order to find the infective particles however, various methods have been attempted.

When antibodies to the prion protein (PrP) are attached to the particles in a sephadex column and infective tissue passed through it, it is found that infective particles also stick to the antibodies (Gabizon et al. 1988). It has also been found that if the infected tissue is subjected to isoelectric focusing, the same band that carries the PrP also carries the infectivity (Ceroni et al. 1990). There is strong evidence that the PrP is infective but this does not rule out the possibility that a small amount of DNA is present inside PrP which is acting as a protective protein.

PrP

This is the prion protein (PrP) associated with SE. A normal form of the protein is found in the membrane of normal nervous tissue cells and is coded by a specific gene. This gene, from chromosome 2 (Sparkes et al. 1986, Prusiner et al. 1987) is highly conserved between strains (Hope et al. 1988) and is altered only between species (Endo et al. 1989, Goldman et al. 1990) and in the GSS syndrome (Collinge et al. 1990). This gene also encodes the scrapie PrP messenger RNA (Cheesebro et al. 1985) and hence the PrP protein (Wietgrefe et al. 1985, Basler et al. 1986, Narang et al. 1988, Borchelt et al. 1990) but it does so in much greater quantities in infected cells. Initially, the protein appears identical to the natural protein, but it becomes modified after production (Basler et al. 1986, Hay et al. 1987, Manuelidis et al. 1987, Caughey et al. 1989). This modification gives rise to the infective form (Endo et al. 1989), and renders the protein resistant to most proteases (Borchelt et al. 1990). When the protein is treated with proteinase K, particles of 27–30 kDa are produced, the structure of which is complex (Barry and Prusiner 1986, Meyer et al. 1986, Bockman and Kingsbury 1988, Hope et al. 1988, Doruru et al. 1989, Serban et al. 1990, Yost et al. 1990), and it varies between species (see above; Kimberlin and Marsh 1975, Bockman et al. 1985) with glycoside residues being added to the molecule (Prusiner et al. 1987, Sklaviadis et al. 1989). Also it appears to vary with scrapie strain (Carlson et al. 1989, Lowenstein et al. 1990), and may vary between strains of animal of the same species (Lopez et al. 1990). In the normal cell the protein is found in the periplasmic membrane and, as such, it has an affinity for joining liposomes or membranes (see above; Prusiner 1982, Gabizon and Prusiner 1990). The modified form however, may be found inside the cell, in the membrane, or as a secretory form (Hay et al.

1987). When antibodies against PrP are made in rabbits to produce polyclonal (Bendheim et al. 1984, Barry et al. 1986, Roberts et al. 1986), or monoclonal antibodies (Barry and Prusiner 1986, Kascsak et al. 1987). These have been used to demonstrate the presence of PrP in the amyloid of some infected tissues (Prusiner et al. 1983, Bockman et al. 1985, de Armond et al. 1985, Roberts et al. 1986, Wiley et al. 1987) and with the scrapie associated fibrils (SAF) (Kimberlin 1989, Liberski et al. 1989a,b) (although this is not always successful (Bode and Diringer 1985)). The use of PrP as an indicator of tissue infection (Farquhar et al. 1989) and its finding in other tissues that are themselves infective but do not contain large amounts of neurological tissue (Kitamoto et al. 1989) have suggested that PrP has indeed a crucial role in infectivity. This issue is at present under fierce scientific debate (de Armond et al. 1989, Manuelidis et al. 1987). Because of these uncertainties, the use of serological reagents to diagnose specific infective agents is fraught with difficulty, but is being studied by several groups.

Prion rods

It has been suggested that PrP will polymerise (de Armond et al. 1985, McKinley et al. 1986) to form prion rods that might be visible under the electron microscope (Prusiner 1982, Prusiner et al. 1983, 1987), similar to SAF, but this is not accepted by all workers.

There are many minor differences in appearance which can be stained by congo red histochemical stains. They possess the same diameter and limited twisting as the shorter rod shaped particles observed in purified preparations of prions (de Armond et al. 1985). Immunological staining has been carried out using antibodies specific for PrP and they themselves have been used to make antibodies (Barry and Prusiner 1986). It has, however, been claimed that there is poor correlation between the presence of prion rods and the site of tissue that is infective. They are not the same as the SAF, which many researchers feel are the infective particles.

Scrapies associated fibrils (SAF)

These are twig-like structures, 12–16 nm in width and 100–500 nm long (Merz et al. 1981, Diringer et al. 1983) seen under the electron microscope (Bode et al. 1985, Liberski et al. 1989a). They are only found in TSE infective tissues (Merz et al. 1984, Hope et al. 1988), and they copurify with infectivity (Bode and Diringer 1985). The fine structure under the electron microscope is different from prion rods (Prusiner et al. 1987, Liberski et al. 1989a,b) but they may be made of a normal or abnormal form of PrP (Hope et al. 1986). Some consider that a form of PrP is present in SAF (Hope et al. 1986) but others disagree (Manuelidis et al. 1987). SAF can be concentrated (Bode et al. 1985), and antibodies made against them (Diringer et al. 1984, Cho 1986, Rubinstein et al. 1986) including monoclonals (Kascsak et al. 1987). Staining techniques generally require the presence of these antibodies (Hope et al. 1986) and the amount of SAF is proportional to the infectivity of the tissue (Merz et al. 1984). No variation in antibodies has yet appeared against different scrapie strains of SAF (Fraser et al. 1989).

The identity of infective agent is still unclear but it is now unlikely that spiroplasmas, AIDS (with which some PrP may immunologically cross-react), or the infective agent in Alzheimers disease are involved. In summary, it is not possible to formulate a unitary hypothesis to account for the nature and mechanism of pathogenicity of the agents causing TSEs. It is likely that some of the conflicting findings will be capable of resolution by further molecular work.

Food and infective dose

Bovine brain was used in many foods, generally meat pies, sausages and beefburgers, until November 1989 when this was banned by the British Government. Brain is defined as 'beef' and not 'beef offal' according to European Community (EC) regulations. Hence, if it was used in the manufacture of beefburgers, the final product could legitimately be known as '100% beef'.

The figures are based on numbers that have been found in other animals with SE. This is an attempt to identify whether potential infective quantities might have been achieved previously.

Bovine brain from animals with clinical BSE (and possibly from those incubating it) is expected to have 10^6–10^{10} infective units (IU) per gram of tissue (Marsh et al. 1969, Hadlow et al. 1974, Kimberlin and Walker 1979, Kimberlin et al. 1983, Prusiner et al. 1985, Kitamoto et al. 1989, Robinson et al. 1990). If it is assumed that the brains of 1000 cows (Tyrrell's most optimistic incidence) were mixed together and one of them had been obtained from an animal with BSE, then the mixture would be expected to contain 10^3–10^7 IU g^{-1}. If 10% of a beefburger was brain tissue then the burger would be expected to contain 10^2–10^6 IU g^{-1}. Animal infection has been shown to take place orally at 4×10^4 IU with a spongiform encephalopathy agent (Kimberlin and Walker 1989). In this case the infective dose would be contained in 0.04–400 g of beefburger. Other experiments have showed, however, an oral infective dose to be 10^9 IU (Prusiner et al. 1985). The lower infective dose is supported by the very wide distribution of BSE in cows and cattle in the UK (Southwood 1989). An infective dose may indeed be much higher but at present this is not known. If the total number of cows infected with BSE was substantially higher than Tyrrell's estimate of 0–1%, then the risks would also increase. The most gloomy prediction of the number of animals infected is 5–10%. The possibility that cows were infected with scrapie in their food could mean that the infective dose for the cow had come from sheep (i.e. crossed the 'species barrier'). One farmer (Winter et al. 1989) reported that 14 of his herd of 500 animals acquired BSE and that each had not had more than 12 kg of protein supplement. It is reasonable to assume that around 1% of this would be brain tissue and that perhaps 1% of the sheep brains would have been infected with scrapie. It should be said at this point that a short survey of Yorkshire sheep farmers showed that only one out of 20 claimed to have seen a case of scrapie in his lifetime, that veterinarians near to Leeds claimed it to be a rare disease and that a well known researcher into the subject (who has asked not to be named) had never seen more than ten cases in a flock. It has been claimed that the number of cases of scrapie in Britain have been increasing but there are no statistics to support this. Hence, we consider that our estimate of 1% of sheep being infected with scrapie is probably an overestimate. If the sheep brain was infected at approximately 10^7 IU g^{-1} (Robinson et al. 1990) then, given these suggestions, his cows would have eaten 2×10^6 IU. For human beings to eat this number of IU from, say, beefburger meat (and hence cross the species barrier from cows to humans), would require them to eat 2 g to 20 kg, assuming that the agent has a specificity to us at all. Such consumption is certainly feasible in practice. Infection with SE prions may be cumulative, i.e. an infective dose can be achieved by taking in small parts over a long period. There is little evidence for this except that there are no antibodies formed in the body against other prion, and hence it might always remain infective.

If this is so then the dose of beefburger mentioned above could have been eaten by many people over the period of a year before November 1989.

Since November 1989, the eating of British beef has continued but under the demands of the British Government, this should not contain any brain, spinal cord or lymphoid tissue (Report 1990). In order for this to be possible the animal may be cut with a saw (Report 1990) so that the brain and spinal cord tissue can be removed (often using suction or irrigation equipment). This may be a dangerous procedure considering that brain tissue has the consistency of blancmange and may be spread over any meat tissue. A piece of bovine central nervous system the size of a sugar grain could convey 10^3–10^7 IU. Also, peripheral nerves have been shown to contain infective prions in goat scrapie and TME (Pattison and Millson 1962, Hadlow et al. 1987) so it is not surprising that meat has been shown to be infective in some animal experiments, although not with BSE as yet (Marsh et al. 1969, Pattison et al. 1972).

The risk of BSE to man

Because of the fragmentary knowledge over the agents responsible for TSEs, it is not possible to make any firm prediction as to whether, or on what scale, man might be infected by the BSE infective agent. There is not even sufficient information to calculate any probabilities and their limits of reliability. Some reports have relied upon the optimistic view that any risk to man is 'remote' (Southwood 1989, Tyrrell 1989). However, the first authors to provide firm reasons for the potential hazard of BSE for man were Holt and Phillips (1988).

In this section, we discuss the information which favours a pessimistic or an optimistic outcome, and give our assessment of the relative certainties of these factors. We ill not be tempted into making an arithmetical prediction.

The study of CJD provides a useful starting point. Formally notified cases are of the order of 30–40 cases annually in the UK. The real numbers are thought to be between 1500 and 9000 (Roberts 1990), the discrepancy arising from the failure to diagnose accurately the nature of fatal dementing illness. If BSE did infect man, it is by no means certain that the resultant disease would be identical to CJD. Degenerative neurological diseases do not always form precisely defined entities. There are some, such as motor neurone diseases, which could also have an infective basis.

There is incontrovertable proof that the infectious agent for CJD can be transmitted from human tissues to experimental animals (*vide supra*). It is virtually certain, therefore, that CJD is caused by the acquisition of that infectious agent. However, it is theoretically possible that the infectious agents associated with or causing CJD evolve *de novo* in an infected individual as a result of genetic disposition or mutation (Goldfarb et al. 1990). If for example, PrPs were the causative agent, and these arose from congenital or environmental affect on a host cell DNA, then fears over the tranmissibility of the BSE agent to man would rescind to some extent; CJD could just possibly not be acquired from meat. The familial incidence of the disease is said to be approximately 15% and might be consistent with this view. However the familial nature of the disease, particularly in Libyan Jews, could be explained by the genes in question conferring a specific disposition to acquiring an exogenous infection. Furthermore, such an apparent genetic basis could result from exposure of members of families to uniform environmental sources such as idiosyncratic diets. It has always been difficult to identify the true biological origin of any infectious agent, whether novel or not. On grounds of probability we must consider that the evolution of such an infective agent *in situ* in so many individuals at any one time must be unlikely.

Moreover, the epidemiology of BSE has produced overwhelming evidence of the existence of an infective agent acquired through the oral route. Whilst it can be argued whether or not BSE is unique to the British Isles, the scale of the epidemic in cattle is manifestly so. Therefore, we believe that the TSEs should be considered to have an infectious basis at the present. Likewise, CJD should therefore be considered an infection. The potential routes of acquisition of the infectious agent – transplacental, mucosal, inhalation, injection, sexual or oral – are all possible. Certainly vertical transmission of scrapie in sheep is known, and vertical transmission of the causal agent for CJD may occur, but at least one other route must be postulated in order to account for the presence of the putative infective agent in so many sporadic cases. Again, the most impressive evidence for the importance of any route of acquisition of these agents comes from BSE in cattle, where the oral route would appear to offer the only plausible explanation. Experimentally, such infections can also be transferred to mice through the oral route (*vide supra*). Whilst there is no proof of this, it would seem likely that oral route in man provides the most likely portal of entry. This is at the very least, the most obvious working hypothesis for most of the cases, but seemingly impossible to prove or disprove. That the spleen is the first organ to be infected in sheep acquiring scrapie experimentally (*vide supra*) is consistent with the view that the infectious agent is capable of penetrating the gastrointestinal tract. Some slight reservation has to be made here because, theoretically, animals fed the infective agent either naturally or experimentally could eliminate it in their faeces, and then acquire the infection through mucosal or skin penetration.

Since all the TSEs have been identified in mammals, then one or more of these must be considered the source of CJD. Until very recently the disease had not been reported in domestic pets. Some contact with say, goats, might on occasion cause the infection. Deer could also be a minor reservoir. The three major sources of animal meat throughout the world must be scrutinised very carefully – i.e. products from cattle, sheep and pigs. The possibility that sheep scrapie might be responsible for CJD has been considered by several workers. Because the incidence of scrapie in sheep varies substantially throughout the world, being highest in Iceland and lowest in New Zealand, it has been possible to look at the varying incidences of the two diseases in a number of countries. No association has been found (e.g. Southwood 1989, Tyrrell 1989). These negative findings do not establish that scrapie never inflicts man, but make an ovine origin most unlikely to be the major source.

Pigs might provide such a reservoir, but a number of factors argue against this. First, pigs apparently do not suffer naturally from SE. Secondly, pig meat is generally eaten when the animal is 5 or 6 months old: that is an age when it would be expected not to be infectious, even if SE did develop subsequently. Thirdly, a high incidence of CJD occurs in Libyan Jews, whose diet presumably excludes pig products.

Thus, through the exclusion of other sources, cattle may be the most likely source of CJD. Consistent with this proposal is the frequency with which beef cattle and cows are slaughtered at the end of their lactation (between 3 and 10 years). Age must be a highly significant factor in the availability of the infectious agent. Urgent research is needed to study the relationship between the consumption of beef products by communities and the coincidence of CJD. If cattle are the sources of CJD, then this implies the presence of an infectious agent long before the recognition of BSE. The first cases of BSE were identified in 1985–6, so it is unlikely that the infectious agent was present in meat products before 1982–3. If the incubation period of CJD is 15–20 years, then current CJD cases cannot be caused by the BSE agent in the 1980s. It is certainly possible that a BSE-like infectious agent could have been present in cattle for many years either without producing clinical infection, or indeed responsible for occasional clinical disease. There are rumours of the existence of cattle suffering a BSE-type disease many years ago in Yorkshire, UK or more recently in other countries and these would be compatible with this view.

The above thesis is of course speculative, but we believe that cattle are the likely major source of the infectious agent for CJD that is acquired through food. There is no proof, but these ideas should prompt further work.

If the putative 1500–9000 cases of CJD in the UK annually have indeed been caused by consumption of beef products some years ago, the potential danger from BSE becomes disturbingly obvious. The most worrying hypothesis must suppose that the infectious agent from BSE-infected cattle is responsible for CJD. If this is the case, the high prevalence of infected animals – estimated at between 1 and 10% – must present a phenomenal danger to man. There is no reason to exclude the possibility that the BSE epidemic represents an 'amplified' natural infection as a result of rendered cattle offal being fed to cattle between 1981 and 1988. This is a different interpretation from the much publicised belief that the sheep scrapie agent was responsible for the BSE epidemic. This proposal was supported by the rearing of increasing numbers of sheep in this country, and an alleged increasing incidence of scrapie in this animal. There is however no direct evidence to support this, illustrating the poor data base that exists for animal infections in this country as a whole. Those who claim that scrapie is the likely source of BSE (e.g. Southwood 1989, Tyrrell 1989) must account for the failure of scrapie to infect cattle previously, despite the sharing of common grazing land for centuries (Morgan 1988). A third possibility has been proposed, namely that the BSE agent represents a mutated scrapie agent whose host range has become altered (Lacey and Dealler, in press).

Beef as a potential hazard to man

The possibility of danger to man from cattle brain and other offal material incorporated into processed items has already been considered (*vide supra*). There is little reason to believe that the agents responsible for transmissible spongiform encephalopathies are found actually within or around muscle fibres, although occasionally the agent has been transferred from muscle (Tables 4 and 5). However, the main danger from beef products is due to the presence of adventitous material, including: peripheral nervous tissue that may contain infectious agent, lymphatics in channels and nodes around beef tissue that may be infectious, and the contamination of the carcase with spinal cord, brain and other 'high-risk' tissues during the processing. In particular, the use of mechanical saws to remove bone could be hazardous in this way.

In discussing the possible effect on man, the most pessimistic view has been taken so far. Any one of the following could substantially reduce the risk.

The first reassurance could come from the failure of the BSE to gain access to the milieu of the human body. It may not adhere to mucous membranes or be able to penetrate gastrointestinal mucosa; it might also be inactivated by blood or proteolytic enzymes in the gut (although this is unlikely). If the BSE agent was heterogeneous in its properties, then at least some of these factors could reduce the risk of entry to the body. The agent may not survive or multiply in the reticulo-endothelial or nervous system. Finally, it might do so so slowly that its adverse effects would not be manifested during the human lifespan.

The concept of an infective dose may not truly apply to the potential of the BSE agent to infect man. It is not known why a certain number of infectious particles of TSEs are required to induce experimental infections. The crucial question remains unanswered. Is a high infectious dose required to provide the certainty of the infectious agent entering a cell at a specific receptor? If this were the case, then the consumption of small amounts of agent on numerous occasions could provide the same risk as consumption of the total number of particles on more than one occasion.

The more optimistic explanation for the requirement of a certain number of particles to generate an experimental infection is that cellular or other immune mechanisms may satisfactorily eliminate the agent up to a critical number at any one time. If this was the case, the repetitive consumption of small numbers of particles over a long term should provide little infectious risk. Exceptions to those would be people with impaired immunity. With either explanation, pregnant women might be most vulnerable.

In conclusion, the scale of the BSE outbreak in the British Isles presents major problems. More research is required to assess the risk to man, and to develop methods for early detection of TSEs before the onset of clinical symptoms. Whilst the evidence that the feed is responsible is compelling, the host range of BSE is not defined. Generally, TSEs are capable of transfer experimentally to about half of the mammals tested.

Addendum

The SE infection of one out of eight pigs which had been parenterally injected with 10% suspensions of BSE in saline after 69 weeks incubation has recently been shown (Dawson et al. 1990). The possibility that pigs fed with BSE infected meal became infected prior to this being banned in September 1990 must be considered (Medrum 1990) and that these animals may be infective to man (Mills 1990).

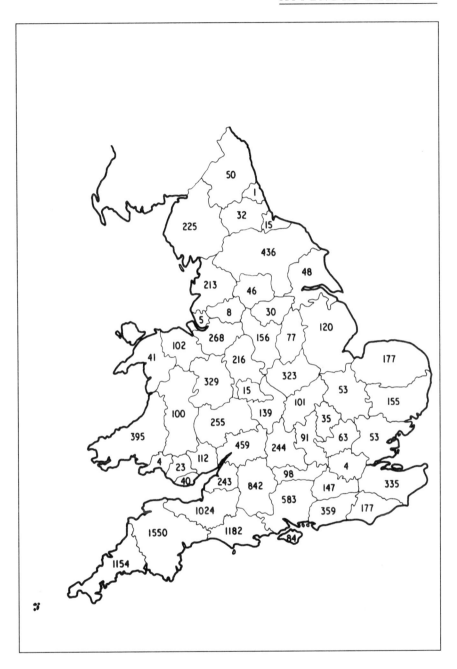

Fig. 1. The number of confirmed cases of BSE in different counties in England and Wales up to 16 April 1990.

INDEX

Richard Lacey is referred to as RL throughout the index

Huddersfield Polytechnic Catering
  Department 26
HUS (Haemolytic Uraemic Syndrome)
  71–2
  caused by poison VTEC
    (*Verocytotoxin*) 63
  cost benefits of preventive
    medicine 66
  cost of dialysis treatments 65–6, 80
  symptoms 62–3
HUSH (Haemolytic Uraemic
  Syndrome Help) 71
  legal action against Department of
    Health and MAFF 71–2
hygiene in the kitchen 189–97
  chopping boards 191
  dishwashers 196
  food processors 196
  freezer 194–5
  hand towels and dishcloths 189–90
  insects 192
  kitchen stove 195
  kitchen surfaces 190
  knives and utensils 190–1
  microwave oven 195
  pets 192, 193
  refrigerator 193–4
  room temperature storage 192
  storage cupboards 192–3
  thermometers for fridge and
    freezer 194
  waste disposal 196–7

Iceland, re-infection of scrapie-free
  sheep 86–7, 241
Institut Pasteur, Paris 33
international ban on UK beef products
  and cattle 227
irradiated food 200–1

Kerr, Dr Kevin 33, 34
kitchen *see* hygiene in the kitchen
Kuru disease 89, 90, 150, 223, 230, 235,
  240, 242–3

Kuru disease *continued*
  effects on brain tissues 88
  incubation period 108–9, 116, 255
  limited to women and children of
    Fore tribe 88, 243
  no antibody reaction 88
  transferable to gibbons and
    monkeys 89
  vertical transmission 89, 135

Lacey, Richard
  advice on cooking eggs 57
  at home *Pl.12*
  attempts by others to discredit
    26–7, 34, 74, 120, 214
    attack by Leeds University
      colleagues 127–9, 130
    early day motion in House of
      Commons 125–6
  book publisher threatened 154–5
  campaign against Septrin 15
  cattle slaughter called for 122
  chairman of Control of Infectious
    Diseases Committee, Leeds
    General Infirmary 151
  concerns at introduction of cook-
    chill to Stanley Royd hospital
    25
  contract at Chapel Allerton
    Hospital 152–3
  death threats 60, 74, 204
  department to be merged with
    Public Health Service
    Laboratory 151, 153
  dispute over numbers of confirmed
    BSE cases 218
  early retirement from Leeds
    University 152, 210
  Evian Award for Medicine and
    Service *Pl.6*
  evidence given to Select Committee
    on Agriculture 133–7, 213–24
  George Orwell Memorial Lecture
    78, 224

National Health Service *continued*
  services privatized 30
Neil, Andrew, editor of the *Sunday
  Times* 215–16

Oprah Winfrey *see* Winfrey, Oprah

palm oil 179
Parker, Doreen, mother of Matthew
  5–10
Parker, Matthew 5–11, 167
  CAT scan 7
  CJD diagnosis 7
  death from new-variant CJD
    10–11
  diet 5–6
  symptoms 6–10
Parliamentary Questions asked on
  behalf of RL
  BSE deaths in Channel Islands and
    Isle of Man 221
  cattle deaths from BSE 220–1
  government sponsored animal
    experiments 219
  procedures for isolating and
    reporting BSE livestock suspects
    221
  testing of sheep scrapie as cause of
    BSE 222–3
Patterson, Professor John 227
Pattison, Professor John, SEAC
  chairman 165, 166
penicillin 16
Pennington, Professor Hugh, inquiry
  into Lanarkshire *E. coli* outbreak
  70–1
personal hygiene 189
pesticides, effects on wildlife 13
Phillips, Lord Justice, chairman of
  new BSE inquiry 203, 207–8
pigs 140, 253, 265, 268
  infected with BSE 140
Porcine Spongiform Encephalopathy
  (PCE) 140

poultry
  cooking methods 185
  factory farming 54
  salmonella infection 21–2, 52, 53,
    58–60, 185
poultry feed, incorporating processed
  poultry remains 54
pregnant women, vulnerable to food
  poisoning 19
Press Association 126, 130
prion diseases
  BSE 94
  different in each species 149, 240,
    250–2
  Kuru 223
  vertical transferability 223
prion rods 261
prions 91, 240, 257–8
  application of genetic engineering
    149–50
  attack brain tissue 92–3, 148
  crossing species barrier 149–50,
    206
  incorporation of host DNA 149,
    252, 258
  indestructible by medical
    techniques or cooking 92, 174,
    195
  long incubation time 92
  unrecognized by immune system
    92, 148
PrP (prion protein) 149, 162, 259–61,
  264
Prusiner, Dr Stanley, discoverer of
  prions 91–3, 102, 148–9
Public Health Laboratory Service 55,
  66, 101, 151
  listeria in cook-chill 31
  merger with RL's department 151,
    153
publications (authored / co-authored
  by RL)
  articles and letters in *The Lancet* 33,
    34–5, 44, 45

279